Keto Diet for Seniors

A Beginner's Guide to Keto Living To Explore the Wonders of the Ketogenic Lifestyle

By

Melinda Francis

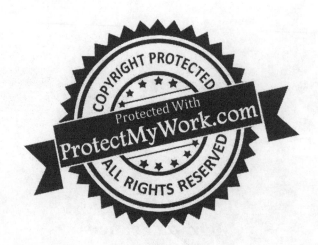

Dear Reader,

Welcome to "Keto Diet For Seniors".

I am Melinda Francis, a nutritionist with a profound commitment to assisting individuals in navigating the challenges of aging with grace and vitality. Drawing from my extensive experience and dedication to promoting healthy living, I have meticulously crafted this comprehensive guide tailored specifically to address the dietary requirements of seniors, particularly those aged over 60.

As someone who understands firsthand the importance of tailored nutrition, I'm excited to share with you a collection of delicious and nutritious recipes designed to support your journey towards better health. Each recipe within this book has been thoughtfully curated to adhere to the principles of the ketogenic diet, while also offering valuable insights into effectively managing health conditions commonly encountered in older age.

I've poured my heart and soul into this book, and I truly believe it has the power to empower you to take charge of your health and well-being. As you explore the pages of this book, I invite you to embark on a culinary adventure with me, embracing positive change and discovering new ways to nourish your body and soul.

Your feedback holds immense significance to me, serving not only to aid my growth as an author but also as a beacon of guidance for fellow readers on their health journeys. I kindly urge you to share your thoughts and experiences by leaving a review on Amazon. Your words will not only bolster my endeavors but also extend a helping hand to others, equipping them to make informed decisions regarding their well-being.

Thank you for choosing "Keto Diet For Seniors".

Together, let's embark on a journey towards a healthier, happier you.

Warm regards,
Melinda Francis

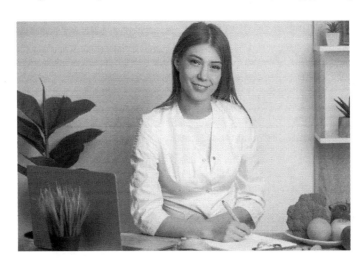

Table of Contents

Introduction...9

Chapter 1: Transformations in Physical Health as We Age..**10**

1.1 Physical Changes Related to Age for Seniors...10

1.2 Commonalities and Differences Between Men and Women in Age-Related Changes............12

1.3 The Impact of the Ketogenic Diet on Aging with Grace...13

Chapter 2: The Ketogenic Diet for Seniors...**14**

2.1 Understanding Ketosis...14

2.2 Achieving Ketosis Safely for Seniors...14

2.3 Varieties of Ketogenic Diets..15

2.4 Tips for Starting and Maintaining the Ketogenic Diet in Older Age.................................19

2.5 Creating a Supportive Network for Seniors on the Ketogenic Journey.............................22

Chapter 3: Pros and Cons of the Ketogenic Diet for Seniors...**24**

3.1 Specific Benefits of the Ketogenic Diet for Seniors...24

3.2 Side Effects of the Ketogenic Diet for Seniors...29

3.3 Managing Ketogenic Diet Side Effects...30

3.4 Embracing the Ketogenic Lifestyle for Seniors..31

3.5 Addressing Common Queries and Concerns..37

3.6 Real-Life Transformations on the Ketogenic Diet...40

Chapter 4: KETO GROCERY LIST..**42**

4.1 Essential Foods for Your Ketogenic Journey...42

4.2 Supplements..44

4.3 Foods To Avoid..45

Chapter 5: Exercise and Fitness for Seniors on a Ketogenic Diet.....................................**47**

5.1 Physical Activity for Healthy Aging...47

5.2 Precautions for Physical Activity in Seniors on the Keto Diet..48

5.3 21-Day Exercise Plan For Women (Compatible with Keto Lifestyle)................................49

5.4 21-Day Exercise Plan For Men (Compatible with Keto Lifestyle)....................................51

5.5 21-Day Exercise Plan For Seniors (Compatible with Keto Lifestyle)................................52

Chapter 6: Keto Recipes For Breakfast..**54**

1. Creamy Avocado and Smoked Salmon Toast...54

2. Blueberry Chia Pudding...55

3. Spinach and Mushroom Breakfast Casserole...55

4. Cauliflower Hash Browns...56

5. Coconut Almond Keto Pancakes..57

6. Cheddar and Chive Keto Biscuits...58

7. Turmeric Scrambled Eggs..59

8. Keto Strawberry Smoothie Bowl..60

9. Bacon-Wrapped Asparagus..60

10. Almond Flour Waffles..61

11. Tomato and Basil Mini Quiches...62

12. Mediterranean Keto Omelette...63

13. Keto Veggie and Cheese Frittata Muffins...63

14. Cinnamon Coconut Porridge...64

15. Savory Keto Crepes..65

16. Pecan Pie Keto Oatmeal..65

17. Coconut Berry Parfait..66

18. Keto Zucchini Bread..67

19. Keto Cinnamon Roll Chaffles..67

20. Greek Yogurt and Walnut Parfait..68

Chapter 7: Keto Recipes For Lunch..69

1. Keto Chicken and Vegetable Stir-Fry..69

2. Spinach and Feta Stuffed Chicken Breast...70

3. Greek-inspired Cucumber and Tomato Salad...70

4. Zucchini Noodles with Pesto and Cherry Tomatoes...71

5. Keto Beef and Broccoli...72

6. Baked Cod with Lemon and Dill...72

7. Asparagus and Prosciutto Wraps...73

8. Eggplant Parmesan...74

9. Shrimp and Cauliflower Rice Stir-Fry...74

10. Cauliflower and Bacon Soup...75

11. Avocado and Tuna Stuffed Bell Peppers...76

12. Keto Turkey and Cranberry Salad...76

13. Keto Cabbage Rolls...77

14. Thai Coconut Chicken Soup..78

15. Spinach and Mushroom Stuffed Pork Chops..78

16. Creamy Garlic Shrimp with Spinach...79

17. Greek Lemon Chicken Soup (Avgolemono Soup)...80

18. Keto BLT Salad..81

19. Spinach and Artichoke Stuffed Chicken...81

20. Salmon and Avocado Salad..82

Chapter 8: Keto Recipes For Dinner..**84**

1. Creamy Spinach and Mushroom Stuffed Pork Tenderloin..84

2. Keto Eggplant Lasagna..84

3. Dijon and Herb Crusted Salmon..85

4. Keto Beef Stroganoff..86

5. Lemon Garlic Shrimp and Zucchini Noodles..86

6. Spicy Cauliflower and Chickpea Curry..87

7. Pesto and Prosciutto-Wrapped Asparagus...88

8. Lemon Butter Baked Cod with Herbed Tomatoes...89

9. Stuffed Zucchini Boats with Ground Turkey...89

10. Creamy Spinach and Artichoke Stuffed Chicken Breasts...90

11. Roasted Garlic and Rosemary Lamb Chops..91

12. Thai-inspired Coconut Shrimp Soup...91

13. Keto Spaghetti Squash Carbonara..92

14. Baked Dijon Mustard and Herb-Crusted Tilapia..93

15. Cabbage and Sausage Stir-Fry...93

16. Keto Pork Chops with Blue Cheese Sauce..94

17. Keto Pesto and Mozzarella Stuffed Chicken..95

18. Lemon Herb Shrimp and Zucchini Noodles...95

19. Beef and Broccoli Stir-Fry with Sesame Seeds..96

20. Stuffed Avocado with Tuna and Olive Tapenade..97

Chapter 9: Keto Recipes For Dessert & Snacks...**98**

1. Coconut Almond Butter Bites..98

2. Pumpkin Spice Keto Cookies..98

3. Matcha Green Tea Fat Bombs...99

4. Keto Peanut Butter Fudge..99

5. Blueberry Almond Keto Granola..100

6. Chocolate Mint Avocado Pudding..101

7. Cinnamon Pecan Keto Brittle..101

8. Vanilla Chia Pudding with Berries..102

9. Keto Cheesecake Bites..103

10. Peanut Butter Chocolate Chip Keto Bars..104

11. Salted Caramel Fat Bombs..104

12. Chocolate Dipped Macadamia Nut Bites...105

13. Coconut Lime Energy Bites...105

14. Keto Tiramisu Fat Bombs..106

15. Keto Cinnamon Donut Holes...107

16. Espresso Keto Truffles...108

17. Keto Mixed Berry Parfait..108

18. Keto Lemon Poppy Seed Muffins...109

19. Cacao Nib and Almond Butter Cups...110

20. Keto Cinnamon Pecan Granola...110

90-Day Keto Meal Plan For Seniors...112

Keto Diet for Seniors Guided Nutrition Tracker...............................126

Guided Roadmap for the Keto Diet...131

Conclusion...132

Introduction

As individuals gracefully transition into their senior years, they encounter a myriad of changes, both externally and internally. This phase of life emphasizes the importance of health, with dietary choices playing a pivotal role. It's during this time that the Ketogenic Diet emerges as a transformative option for seniors, offering a well-researched approach to nutrition.

As a seasoned nutritionist, I've had the privilege of guiding countless seniors towards better health. Among the array of dietary strategies available, the Ketogenic Diet stands out for its potential benefits for individuals in their later years. While commonly associated with weight management, the keto diet's emphasis on low-carbohydrate, high-fat consumption holds promise in enhancing mental clarity and overall vitality.

In the chapters ahead, we will delve into the nuances of the Ketogenic Diet tailored specifically for seniors. We'll explore its potential benefits for both men and women, with a keen focus on addressing the unique nutritional needs of older adults. Throughout the book, we'll make important distinctions between the sexes concerning the ketogenic diet, recognizing the importance of personalized approaches to health.

However, embarking on this journey requires both enthusiasm and caution. While the Ketogenic Diet offers numerous advantages, it's essential to navigate it safely, considering potential risks and individual health conditions.

This book serves as your companion on the path to better health, empowering you with knowledge and practical insights to make informed choices about nutrition. You'll find meticulously crafted sections including a comprehensive grocery list, practical tips for seamlessly integrating the ketogenic lifestyle, specially tailored recipes, and a structured meal plan. Additionally, we'll provide exercise plans designed for both couples and individuals, as well as separate plans tailored to the unique needs of senior men and women.

So, let's embark on this journey together, unlocking the potential of the Ketogenic Diet for seniors and discovering a path to a healthier and more vibrant life, irrespective of age or gender.

Chapter 1: Transformations in Physical Health as We Age

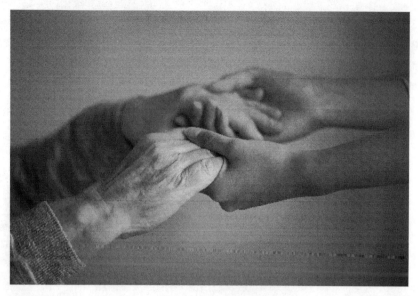

As we journey through life, our bodies undergo significant transformations, particularly as we advance in age. These changes, both physiological and psychological, play a crucial role in shaping our health and well-being.

1.1 Physical Changes Related to Age for Seniors

As individuals enter their senior years, it's natural for the body to undergo a series of physical changes. One notable change is the gradual loss of muscle mass and strength, a phenomenon known as sarcopenia. This decline in muscle mass can lead to decreased mobility, increased risk of falls, and reduced overall functionality. Another common age-related change is alterations in bone density, often resulting in osteoporosis or osteopenia. Weaker bones increase the risk of fractures and can significantly impact an individual's quality of life. Additionally, seniors may experience changes in metabolism and hormonal balance, which can affect weight management and overall energy levels. Hormonal fluctuations, particularly in women during menopause, can contribute to changes in body composition and distribution of fat. Furthermore, aging often brings about changes in sensory perception, including vision and hearing impairments. These changes can impact dietary choices and food preferences, necessitating adjustments in nutritional intake. It's essential to recognize that while these physical changes are a natural part of the aging process, proactive measures can be taken to mitigate their impact. Through a combination of balanced nutrition, regular exercise, and appropriate medical care, seniors can maintain optimal health and vitality well into their later years.

Let's delve deeper into all these changes we've discussed:

Loss of Muscle Mass and Strength. Sarcopenia, the gradual loss of muscle mass and strength, is a common occurrence as individuals age. This decline in muscle mass not only affects physical appearance but also impacts functionality and mobility. Seniors experiencing sarcopenia may find it challenging to perform daily activities, leading to a decrease in overall quality of life.

Maintaining muscle mass through resistance training exercises and adequate protein intake is crucial for mitigating the effects of sarcopenia and preserving functional independence.

Changes in Bone Density. Age-related changes in bone density, often resulting in osteoporosis or osteopenia, pose significant health risks for seniors. Weakened bones are more susceptible to fractures, especially in weight-bearing areas such as the hips, spine, and wrists. Osteoporosis can lead to debilitating injuries and a loss of independence. Calcium and vitamin D supplementation, along with weight-bearing exercises like walking or resistance training, are essential for maintaining bone health and reducing the risk of fractures in older adults.

Metabolic and Hormonal Changes. Seniors may experience alterations in metabolism and hormonal balance, affecting weight management and energy levels. Metabolic rate naturally declines with age, leading to decreased calorie expenditure and potential weight gain if dietary habits remain unchanged. Hormonal fluctuations, particularly in women during menopause, can further exacerbate changes in body composition, leading to increased abdominal fat deposition and a higher risk of metabolic disorders like diabetes and cardiovascular disease. Adopting a balanced diet rich in lean proteins, whole grains, fruits, and vegetables, combined with regular physical activity, can help regulate metabolism and support overall health and well-being in older adults.

Digestive Changes. The digestive system can become less efficient with age, leading to issues like constipation and decreased nutrient absorption. A well-designed diet can help alleviate these concerns.

Immune System. Aging can weaken the immune system's response, making older individuals more susceptible to infections. Proper nutrition plays a crucial role in supporting immune function.

Chronic Health Conditions. With age, the risk of chronic health conditions like diabetes, heart disease, and hypertension tends to rise. Dietary strategies like the Ketogenic Diet can influence these conditions positively.

Sensory Changes. Aging often brings about changes in sensory perception, including vision and hearing impairments. Visual acuity tends to decline with age, making tasks like reading, driving, and navigating unfamiliar environments more challenging. Hearing loss, another common age-related change, can lead to social isolation and communication difficulties. These sensory changes can impact dietary choices and food preferences, necessitating adjustments in nutritional intake. Seniors with vision or hearing impairments may benefit from assistive devices or modifications to their environment to enhance independence and quality of life.

Skin Changes. The skin tends to lose its elasticity, becoming thinner and more prone to wrinkles with age. Emphasizing the importance of sun protection and skincare is crucial to preserving skin health in advanced age.

Cardiovascular System. Arteries can harden with age, increasing the risk of heart diseases. Adopting a balanced diet and making regular physical activity a part of your routine can both help assist in keeping your cardiovascular system in good health.

Cognitive Changes. Aging may lead to cognitive changes, including mild memory decline in some individuals. However, it is vital to highlight that the brain has the capacity to adapt and improve through cognitive training.

Lung Function. Lung capacity may decrease with age, making it more important to avoid smoking and maintain an active lifestyle.

By addressing these changes with proactive measures such as proper nutrition, regular exercise, and medical care, seniors can mitigate the impact of aging on their physical health and maintain vitality throughout their later years.

1.2 Commonalities and Differences Between Men and Women in Age-Related Changes

We know that by now. As individuals age, both men and women undergo a series of physiological transformations, yet certain nuances distinguish their experiences. As we have already said, one notable commonality is the gradual decline in muscle mass and strength, known as sarcopenia, which affects both genders. However, research suggests that men tend to experience a slower rate of muscle loss compared to women, potentially due to differences in hormonal profiles and lifestyle factors. Similarly, changes in bone density, leading to conditions like osteoporosis, affect both men and women as they age.

However, women are generally at a higher risk of developing osteoporosis due to factors such as hormonal fluctuations during menopause and lower peak bone mass compared to men. This discrepancy underscores the importance of tailored approaches to bone health for each gender. Metabolic and hormonal changes also manifest differently between men and women. While both genders may experience a decline in metabolic rate with age, hormonal fluctuations, particularly during menopause, can significantly impact women's body composition and weight management. Men, on the other hand, may be more prone to visceral fat accumulation and metabolic syndrome, increasing their risk of cardiovascular disease and diabetes. Furthermore, sensory changes, such as declines in vision and hearing, can vary in severity and onset between men and women.

While age-related vision impairments like cataracts and macular degeneration affect both genders, studies suggest that men may be more susceptible to hearing loss as they age.

Understanding these commonalities and differences is essential for tailoring interventions and healthcare strategies to meet the unique needs of men and women as they age. By addressing these age-related changes proactively and holistically, individuals can optimize their health and well-being, regardless of gender.

1.3 The Impact of the Ketogenic Diet on Aging with Grace

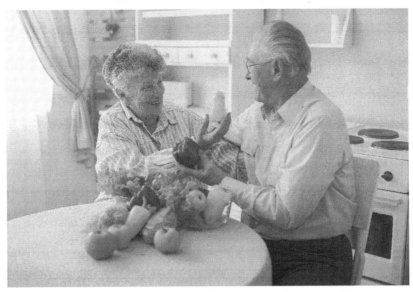

The ketogenic diet, commonly known as the keto diet, has garnered considerable attention recently for its potential advantages in promoting healthy aging. This dietary regimen emphasizes the consumption of high-fat, low-carbohydrate foods, prompting the body to enter a state of ketosis. The role of the ketogenic diet in aging gracefully encompasses various facets of physical and cognitive well-being. Particularly beneficial for older adults is its potential to support weight management. As individuals age, maintaining a healthy weight becomes progressively challenging, and excess weight can lead to various health concerns. The keto diet's capacity to facilitate weight loss by burning stored fats can prove advantageous for seniors seeking to shed extra pounds.

Furthermore, the ketogenic diet has shown promise in enhancing cardiovascular health. By reducing carbohydrate intake and increasing the consumption of heart-healthy fats, it may help mitigate the risk of cardiovascular diseases that become more prevalent with age. Cognitive function is another pivotal aspect of healthy aging. While more research is required in this domain, some studies suggest that the keto diet may possess neuroprotective properties, potentially augmenting brain health and cognitive function in older individuals.

Moreover, the keto diet's impact on energy levels and vitality in seniors warrants consideration. By furnishing a consistent energy source through fats, it may help alleviate fatigue and support an active lifestyle.

In summary, the ketogenic diet holds promise as a dietary approach for aging gracefully. Its potential benefits in weight management, cardiovascular health, cognitive function, and overall vitality make it a subject of significant interest for seniors aiming to age with grace and maintain a high quality of life.

Chapter 2: The Ketogenic Diet for Seniors

2.1 Understanding Ketosis

Ketosis lies at the core of the ketogenic diet, and it's vital to comprehend how this metabolic state functions. Ketosis occurs when the body shifts from utilizing carbohydrates as its primary source of energy to relying on fats instead. This transition is initiated by a significant reduction in carbohydrate intake, prompting the synthesis of molecules known as ketones. Ketones serve as an alternative fuel source, particularly for the brain and other vital organs. For seniors embarking on the keto diet, ketosis offers several benefits. Firstly, it facilitates weight management by promoting the breakdown of stored fat for energy—a valuable asset as aging often brings about changes in metabolism and increased fat accumulation. Secondly, ketosis helps regulate appetite, potentially aiding in portion control and calorie management. Lastly, ketones themselves may possess neuroprotective properties, supporting cognitive health in older adults. Attaining ketosis necessitates careful control of macronutrient intake, primarily carbohydrates. Typically, a ketogenic diet restricts carbohydrate consumption to approximately 20-50 grams per day. This low-carb approach forces the body to deplete its glycogen reserves and transition into ketosis. The duration required to enter ketosis varies among individuals but generally ranges from a few days to a week. Several common signs indicate the onset of ketosis, including increased thirst, alterations in breath odor, and diminished appetite. Additionally, many individuals experience initial weight loss, primarily due to water loss. It's important to note that individuals may exhibit varying sensitivities to ketosis, and not everyone will display the aforementioned indicators.

2.2 Achieving Ketosis Safely for Seniors

For seniors, achieving and maintaining ketosis should be done with care. Here's how:

- ✓ **Dietary Fat Intake:** Seniors should prioritize healthy fats, like avocados, nuts, and olive oil, while avoiding unhealthy trans fats. This shift in fat intake helps the body transition into ketosis.

- ✓ **Protein Moderation:** Protein intake should be moderate. Consuming excessive protein can lead to gluconeogenesis, where protein converts into glucose, potentially disrupting ketosis. It's vital to strike the right balance.

- ✓ **Carbohydrate Restriction:** Limiting carb intake is crucial. Seniors should focus on low-carb vegetables like leafy greens and cruciferous vegetables while avoiding high-carb foods like grains and sugary treats.

- ✓ **Hydration:** Staying well-hydrated is vital, especially for seniors, as they may be more prone to dehydration. Water helps the body process ketones and supports overall health.

- ✓ **Electrolyte Balance:** Ketosis can affect electrolyte levels. Seniors should ensure an adequate intake of sodium, potassium, and magnesium to prevent imbalances.

- ✓ **Medical Supervision:** It's advisable for seniors to consult a healthcare professional before starting a ketogenic diet, especially if they have underlying health conditions or take medications. Medical supervision ensures safety.

- ✓ **Gradual Transition:** Seniors should gradually transition into ketosis, allowing the body to adapt. This approach reduces the risk of adverse effects.

- ✓ **Monitoring Ketone Levels:** It's crucial for beginners in the ketogenic journey, especially seniors, to have a clear understanding of monitoring ketone levels. Ketone levels indicate whether the body has entered a state of ketosis, which is fundamental for the success of the ketogenic diet. Ketosis is a metabolic state where the body primarily uses ketones, which are produced from fat breakdown, as its energy source instead of carbohydrates. To ensure that ketosis is achieved safely and maintained effectively, regular monitoring is key.

What are Ketone Meters? Ketone meters are user-friendly devices designed to measure the concentration of ketones in the blood. They offer a straightforward way to track your progress on the ketogenic diet. Here's how they work:

- ✓ **Pricking the Finger:** To use a ketone meter, a tiny drop of blood is obtained by pricking the fingertip with a lancet. This process is relatively painless and minimally invasive.

- ✓ **Ketone Strips:** The blood drop is then placed on a specialized ketone strip that is inserted into the meter. These strips contain enzymes that react with the ketones in the blood.

- ✓ **Reading the Results:** Within secs, the meter displays the concentration of ketones in the blood, typically measured in millimoles per liter (mmol/L). This reading provides immediate feedback on whether you are in ketosis.

By regularly using ketone meters, beginners can gain valuable insights into their progress and make informed decisions about their dietary choices. It's an vital tool for ensuring that the ketogenic diet is working effectively and safely, especially for seniors who are new to this approach.

2.3 Varieties of Ketogenic Diets

Within the realm of ketogenic diets, there exist several variations, each offering its unique approach and benefits. As seniors embark on their ketogenic journey, understanding these diverse types is crucial to select the one that aligns best with their needs and preferences. Here, we'll explore the different kinds of keto diets, elaborating on each one comprehensively.

1. Standard Ketogenic Diet (SKD)

The Standard Ketogenic Diet (SKD) stands as the most common and widely practiced form of the ketogenic diet. It entails a high consumption of fats, a moderate intake of protein, and a minimal intake of carbohydrates. The typical macronutrient ratio comprises approximately 70-75% fats, 20-25% protein, and 5-10% carbohydrates. SKD proves suitable for those seeking to achieve and maintain ketosis effectively.

Let's examine the advantages and disadvantages of SKD for seniors:

Advantages for Seniors

- ✓ **Steady Weight Management:** SKD can aid seniors in maintaining a healthy weight. The low carbohydrate intake encourages the body to utilize fat for energy, potentially facilitating weight loss or weight maintenance, a crucial aspect of senior health.

- ✓ **Blood Sugar Control:** SKD may contribute to regulating blood sugar levels, particularly beneficial for individuals grappling with age-related insulin resistance or diabetes.

- ✓ **Brain Health:** The high-fat content in SKD provides a rich source of brain-boosting nutrients. For seniors, this can support cognitive function and potentially mitigate the risk of age-related cognitive decline.

Disadvantages for Seniors

- ✗ **Potential Nutrient Deficiencies:** SKD may occasionally lead to nutrient deficiencies, particularly in essential vitamins and minerals. For seniors, it's imperative to ensure proper micronutrient intake to bolster overall health.

- ✗ **Digestive Challenges:** Some seniors may encounter digestive issues during the transition to SKD due to altered fiber intake. Adequate fiber and hydration are crucial to alleviate potential discomfort.

- ✗ **Medication Adjustments:** Seniors who are on medications should consult with a healthcare provider before commencing SKD, as adjustments to medication may be necessary owing to metabolic changes

2. Targeted Ketogenic Diet (TKD)

The Targeted Ketogenic Diet (TKD) is tailored for individuals who engage in regular physical activities or workouts. It permits a slightly higher intake of carbohydrates around the time of exercise to supply additional energy. This approach enables athletes or active seniors to sustain their performance while remaining in ketosis.

Advantages for Seniors

- ✓ **Enhanced Physical Performance:** KD's increased carb intake around workouts can offer a surge of energy, facilitating participation in physical activities for seniors without experiencing fatigue.

- ✓ **Muscle Preservation:** For active seniors, TKD can aid in preserving muscle mass, essential for maintaining strength and mobility as one ages.

- ✓ **Improved Recovery:** The supplementary carbohydrates can contribute to post-exercise recovery, diminishing the likelihood of muscle soreness and fostering overall well-being.

Disadvantages for Seniors

- ✗ **Precision Required:** TKD demands precise timing of carbohydrate consumption around workouts. For some older individuals, maintaining this level of precision may prove challenging.

- **×** **Carb Tolerance:** Seniors may exhibit varying levels of carbohydrate tolerance. Monitoring blood sugar levels closely and consulting with a qualified medical practitioner is essential to determine the appropriate amount of carbohydrate intake.

- **×** **Individual Variability:** The efficacy of TKD can vary among seniors. It may not be suitable for everyone, necessitating an assessment of whether it aligns with one's fitness objectives and the body's response.

3. Cyclical Ketogenic Diet (CKD)

The Cyclical Ketogenic Diet (CKD) involves alternating between periods of strict keto (low-carb) and higher-carb intake. For instance, individuals may adhere to a strict keto diet for five days followed by two days of increased carbohydrate consumption. CKD offers increased flexibility and is often favored by those who struggle to adhere to a standard keto diet over the long term.

Advantages for Seniors

- **✓** **Dietary Variety:** CKD permits a broader range of food options, including carbohydrate-rich choices during the carb-loading phase. This variety may appeal to seniors seeking more diverse meal selections.

- **✓** **Metabolic Flexibility:** CKD assists older individuals in maintaining metabolic flexibility, crucial for adapting to dietary variations and diverse energy requirements.

- **✓** **Sustainability:** The cyclical pattern of CKD offers respite from strict keto, which some seniors may find challenging to maintain over the long term.

Disadvantages for Seniors

- **×** **Carb Management:** Proper management of carbohydrate intake during the carb-loading phase is essential. Seniors must meticulously monitor their carbohydrate consumption to avoid potential fluctuations in blood sugar levels.

- **×** **Individual Variability:** The effectiveness of CKD may vary from one person to another. It's imperative for seniors to evaluate how their bodies respond to the alternating phases of keto and carb-loading.

- **×** **Consultation Required:** Before embarking on CKD, seniors should seek guidance from healthcare professionals or nutritionists to ensure it aligns with their specific health objectives and dietary requirements.

4. High-Protein Ketogenic Diet

This variation maintains a high fat intake but allows for increased protein consumption. It may suit seniors who prioritize muscle maintenance or are concerned about meeting their protein needs while adhering to a keto diet.

Advantages for Seniors

- **✓** **Muscle Maintenance:** The High-Protein Ketogenic Diet permits a higher protein intake, beneficial for seniors aiming to preserve muscle mass. It helps prevent muscle loss and promotes overall strength.

- ✓ **Satiety:** Elevated protein intake enhances feelings of fullness and satiety, which can be advantageous for seniors who struggle with overeating or cravings.

- ✓ **Nutrient Density:** Emphasizing protein-rich foods can supply essential nutrients, particularly beneficial for seniors striving to meet their dietary requirements effectively.

Disadvantages for Seniors

- ✗ **Potential for Kidney Strain:** High protein intake may strain the kidneys, particularly in individuals with pre-existing kidney issues. Seniors should consult healthcare professionals to ensure their kidneys can handle the increased protein load.

- ✗ **Digestive Challenges:** Older adults may experience digestive sensitivities, and a high-protein diet might exacerbate these issues, leading to digestive discomfort in some cases.

- ✗ **Risk of Excess Calories:** While protein promotes satiety, seniors must monitor their calorie intake. Excessive calorie consumption, even from protein, can contribute to weight gain.

5. Vegetarian or Vegan Ketogenic Diet

For individuals who prefer a plant-based approach, the vegetarian or vegan ketogenic diet substitutes animal products with plant-based fats and protein sources while adhering to low carbohydrate intake. It necessitates meticulous planning to ensure adequate nutrient intake.

Advantages for Seniors

- ✓ **Weight Management:** The Vegetarian or Vegan Ketogenic Diet can aid in weight management, a common concern for seniors. By restricting carbohydrates and emphasizing plant-based fats and proteins, it can contribute to weight control.

- ✓ **Heart Health:** Reducing reliance on animal products can promote heart health. A plant-based approach lowers saturated fat intake, potentially mitigating the risk of heart-related issues.

- ✓ **Blood Sugar Control:** For individuals with diabetes or those monitoring blood sugar levels, a low-carb vegetarian or vegan keto diet can assist in managing blood sugar levels effectively.

Disadvantages for Seniors

- ✗ **Nutrient Planning:** Following a vegetarian or vegan keto diet requires meticulous nutrient planning to ensure seniors obtain essential vitamins and minerals. This may entail supplementation or a well-rounded selection of plant-based foods.

- ✗ **Protein Intake:** Seniors must maintain adequate protein intake for muscle and bone health. A plant-based keto diet may necessitate extra attention to protein sources to ensure sufficiency.

- ✗ **Digestive Changes:** Aging often brings about changes in digestion. A diet rich in plant-based fats and proteins may not be suitable for all seniors and can potentially lead to digestive discomfort.

6. Lazy Keto

Lazy Keto simplifies macronutrient tracking by primarily focusing on carbohydrate intake, offering a more accessible approach compared to other forms of the keto diet.

Advantages for Seniors

✓ **Simplicity:** Lazy Keto streamlines macronutrient tracking by prioritizing carbohydrate intake. This simplicity can make it more approachable for seniors who may find detailed tracking challenging.

✓ **Potential Weight Loss:** By reducing carb intake, Lazy Keto may facilitate weight loss, beneficial for older adults seeking weight management.

Disadvantages for Seniors

✗ **Lack of Precision:** Lazy Keto may not yield the same precise results as other ketogenic variations. Seniors aiming for specific health outcomes, such as blood sugar management or addressing medical conditions, may not achieve desired results as effectively.

✗ **Nutrient Balance:** While Lazy Keto simplifies carb tracking, seniors must not overlook overall nutrient balance. It's crucial to ensure adequate intake of essential vitamins and minerals for optimal health.

✗ **Individual Variability:** Seniors have diverse nutritional needs, and Lazy Keto may not cater to these individual variations effectively.

2.4 Tips for Starting and Maintaining the Ketogenic Diet in Older Age

Embarking on the ketogenic journey in your golden years can bring about transformative health benefits, but it's essential to approach it with careful consideration and preparation. As you delve into the ketogenic lifestyle, keep in mind these practical tips. I am aware that I have repeatedly stated it, but firstly, consult with a healthcare professional before making any significant dietary changes, especially if you have underlying health conditions or are taking medications. Their guidance can ensure the diet aligns with your individual health goals and needs. Secondly, ease into the ketogenic diet gradually, allowing your body time to adjust to the new way of eating. Start by gradually reducing your carbohydrate intake while increasing healthy fats and lean proteins. This gradual transition can help minimize any potential side effects and optimize your chances of success. Additionally, prioritize whole, nutrient-dense foods to meet your nutritional needs adequately. Include plenty of non-starchy vegetables, lean meats, fatty fish, nuts, seeds, and healthy oils in your meals to ensure you're getting a wide array of essential vitamins, minerals, and antioxidants. Stay hydrated by drinking plenty of water throughout the day, as dehydration can exacerbate certain side effects of the ketogenic diet, such as constipation or fatigue. Finally, listen to your body and adjust your approach as needed. Pay attention to how different foods make you feel and make adjustments accordingly. Remember, the ketogenic diet is not one-size-fits-all, and what works for one person may not work for another. Be patient with yourself and celebrate small victories along the way as you work towards optimal health and vitality in your senior years.

With diligence, perseverance, and a positive mindset, you can successfully navigate the ketogenic journey and reap its many benefits well into your golden years. As we customize the ketogenic diet for older women, it's crucial to understand that dietary needs can vary with age. While highly beneficial for seniors, the ketogenic diet requires certain adaptations to suit their unique requirements.

Let's now delve into practical tips for starting the ketogenic diet as a senior.

- ✓ **Macronutrient Ratios:** Your body may have different macronutrient needs compared to younger individuals. While the standard keto diet typically consists of approximately 70-75% fat, 20-25% protein, and 5-10% carbohydrates, these ratios might need some modifications for seniors like yourself. A few may find it beneficial to mildly increase protein intake to maintain muscle mass and overall health.

- ✓ **Micronutrients:** Seniors often require more attention to micronutrients like calcium, vitamin D, and fiber. Incorporating keto-friendly foods rich in these nutrients is vital for your well-being. For example, dairy products, leafy greens, and certain nuts can provide calcium, while fatty fish and egg yolks offer vitamin D.

- ✓ **Hydration:** Drinking enough water is vital for healthy digestion. Ensure you stay well-hydrated throughout the day to support your digestive system.

- ✓ **Slowly Increase Fiber Intake:** To prevent digestive discomfort, slowly incorporate fiber-rich foods into your diet. Foods like leafy greens, avocados, and low-carb vegetables can provide the fiber you need.

- ✓ **Probiotic Foods:** Including probiotic-rich foods like yogurt or kefir in your diet can promote a healthy gut. These foods contain beneficial bacteria that can aid in digestion.

- ✓ **Chew Your Food:** Take your time when eating and chew your food thoroughly. This simple practice can make digestion more comfortable and efficient.

- ✓ **Monitor Fatty Foods:** While fats are a significant part of the ketogenic diet, be mindful of the types and amounts of fats you consume. A few individuals may experience digestive issues with very high-fat meals, so adjust as needed.

- ✓ **Supplementation:** Depending on your individual needs and medical advice, you may benefit from dietary supplements. Common supplements like calcium, vitamin D, and B vitamins can support your overall well-being.

- ✓ **Portion Control:** Managing portion sizes plays a significant role in weight management and overall health, especially for seniors like yourself. Practice portion control to prevent overeating, which can lead to unwanted weight gain.

- ✓ **Balanced Variety:** Emphasize the importance of a well-balanced, varied diet. Include a range of keto-friendly foods to ensure you receive vital nutrients.

- ✓ **Personal Preferences:** Consider your taste preferences and dietary requirements when planning meals. Customizing your meals can make the diet more enjoyable and sustainable.

- ✓ **Nutrient-Dense Choices:** Opt for nutrient-dense foods rich in vitamins and minerals to support your bone health, heart health, and overall well-being.

- ✓ **Avoid Extreme Restrictions:** While the ketogenic diet can be beneficial, it's important not to overly restrict certain food groups or nutrients. Striking a balanced approach ensures you receive vital nutrients.

- ✓ **Regular Health Check-Ups:** It's vital for you, as a woman over 70 following a ketogenic diet, to schedule regular health check-ups with your healthcare provider. These check-ups help monitor your overall health and ensure that the diet aligns perfectly with your specific needs.

- ✓ **Medication Adjustments:** If you are taking medications, be aware that the ketogenic diet can sometimes affect their effectiveness. Discuss any necessary adjustments with your healthcare provider.

- ✓ **Adjustments Based on Your Responses:** Your response to the ketogenic diet may differ from others. A few may enter ketosis more simply than others, while some may require slight modifications to their macronutrient ratios. Listen to your body and make necessary adjustments based on your individual responses.

Social and emotional support

As seniors embark on the keto diet journey, it's essential to acknowledge the unique challenges they might face. Social and emotional obstacles can arise, but there are practical strategies to navigate these challenges effectively:

- ✓ **Share Your Goals:** Communicate your dietary goals with your close circle of friends and family. By explaining why you've chosen the ketogenic diet to support your health, you can garner understanding and encouragement from your loved ones.

- ✓ **Plan Ahead:** Prioritize planning your meals in advance when attending social gatherings. If possible, communicate your dietary preferences to the host to ensure your needs are accommodated.

- ✓ **Maintain Positivity:** Focus on the positive aspects of your dietary changes, such as improved health and vitality. Cultivating a positive mindset can bolster your motivation and resilience along the way.

- ✓ **Join Supportive Communities:** Engaging with supportive communities can significantly enhance your ketogenic journey, providing invaluable resources, encouragement, and shared experiences.

- ✓ **Practice Self-Compassion:** Embrace self-compassion throughout your dietary journey. Allow yourself the occasional indulgence without guilt, and remember that progress is a gradual process.

- ✓ **Embrace Mindfulness:** Incorporate mindfulness into your eating habits. Pay attention to your body's hunger and fullness cues, savor each bite mindfully, and relish the sensory experience of eating.

2.5 Creating a Supportive Network for Seniors on the Ketogenic Journey

For seniors, especially women over 70, embarking on the path to better health through mindful eating is greatly facilitated by the presence of a strong and supportive community. Such a network goes beyond mere gatherings; it fosters an environment where individuals can freely exchange their experiences, triumphs, and challenges. Within these communities, the wealth of wisdom accumulated over a lifetime becomes a valuable resource for all members, providing emotional support, motivation, and a profound sense of belonging essential for nurturing healthier habits. One effective way to connect with like-minded individuals is through online communities, particularly Facebook groups dedicated to the ketogenic diet. Groups such as "Keto for Seniors," "Keto Over 60," or "Ketogenic Living" serve as virtual hubs where seniors can gather to share their journeys, offer advice, and exchange practical tips and recipe ideas. These online platforms provide a space where members can find camaraderie and understanding as they navigate their dietary paths. In addition to online communities, seniors can seek out local meetup groups or clubs focused on ketogenic living. Platforms like Meetup.com or community bulletin boards often list gatherings and events tailored to keto enthusiasts. By participating in local meetups, seniors can enjoy face-to-face interactions with others who share similar dietary goals. Engaging with local communities not only fosters supportive friendships but also opens doors to group activities and shared meals, further enriching the ketogenic experience. Furthermore, exploring national organizations or associations dedicated to promoting ketogenic living can provide seniors with additional support and resources. Organizations like the Ketogenic Diet Foundation or the Nutrition Coalition offer educational materials, forums, and events specifically designed to address the unique needs of seniors on a ketogenic lifestyle. Connecting with national organizations allows seniors to access expert advice, stay updated on research, and join a broader community of individuals committed to supporting each other on their ketogenic journeys. As I said before, by actively participating in supportive networks, seniors can enhance their ketogenic experience, find encouragement, and stay motivated on their journey toward improved health and well-being.

Building Your Network

Creating a network that truly supports and enhances your ketogenic journey requires a thoughtful approach. Here are some essential steps to consider:

- ✓ **Identify Your Contacts:** Begin by compiling a list of your acquaintances, both personal and professional. Your existing contacts serve as the foundation of your network.

- ✓ **Join Relevant Groups:** Seek out groups or organizations that resonate with your interests and goals. Participating in these communities can help you connect with individuals who share similar aspirations.

- ✓ **Online Networking:** Utilize online platforms such as LinkedIn to broaden your connections. Online networking enables you to engage with professionals from diverse backgrounds and geographical locations. Platforms like Facebook offer opportunities to join groups related to your interests or hobbies, facilitating connections with like-minded individuals.

Additionally, video conferencing tools like Zoom and Skype are excellent for virtual face-to-face meetings, enabling seniors to stay connected with loved ones and participate in virtual discussions and events. Various websites host forums where seniors can exchange ideas, seek advice, and share experiences, such as SeniorNet, AARP Community, and Reddit's "Over 60" subreddit. Don't hesitate to seek assistance from family members or friends, particularly those proficient in technology, to help set up your online profiles and navigate these platforms effectively.

✓ **Effective Communication:** Cultivating a supportive network entails engaging in meaningful conversations, sharing experiences, and actively listening to others.

✓ **Reciprocity:** Remember that networking involves giving and receiving support. By offering assistance and support to your network members, you're likely to receive reciprocal help in return.

✓ **Consistency:** Consistency is key to network building. Dedicate regular time each week to networking activities, whether it's reaching out to contacts via email, attending networking events, or participating in online discussions.

✓ **Professional Development:** Prioritize your professional growth by attending workshops, seminars, and conferences. These events provide opportunities to expand your network, acquire new knowledge, and gain valuable insights.

✓ **Mentoring:** Consider becoming a mentor or seeking mentorship within your network. Mentorship relationships can be mutually beneficial, offering guidance, support, and valuable insights.

Engaging in community participation and involvement offers numerous benefits:

✓ **Sense of Belonging:** Active involvement in communities fosters a sense of belonging, reducing feelings of isolation and loneliness among individuals.

✓ **Psychosocial Health:** Community engagement can enrich lives and contribute to improved psychosocial health, positively impacting mental well-being and emotional health.

✓ **Emotional Well-Being:** Building meaningful relationships within a community is integral to emotional well-being, contributing to a positive outlook on life.

✓ **Social Support:** Communities serve as vital support systems where individuals can give and receive social support, reducing stress, promoting independence, and shaping identities.

✓ **Health Benefits:** Participation in community activities and senior centers can lead to enhanced health and overall well-being among older adults. Engaging in community-based initiatives empowers individuals to take charge of their health, fostering self-efficacy and empowerment.

Chapter 3: Pros and Cons of the Ketogenic Diet for Seniors

3.1 Specific Benefits of the Ketogenic Diet for Seniors

In this chapter of 'Keto Diet For Seniors,' we'll explore the numerous benefits that the ketogenic diet can offer to seniors. It's essential to understand that every individual's journey with the ketogenic diet is unique, and while it may present certain challenges, it also brings forth numerous benefits, especially for older adults.

1. Weight Management and Fat Loss

As we journey through life, maintaining a healthy weight becomes increasingly important, especially as we age. The ketogenic diet presents itself as a valuable tool in this regard, offering seniors a pathway to effective weight management and fat loss while preserving essential muscle mass. The ketogenic diet operates on the principle of reducing carbohydrate intake, which triggers a metabolic state known as ketosis. In ketosis, the body shifts its primary source of fuel from carbohydrates to fats and ketones. This metabolic switch enhances the body's ability to burn fat efficiently, facilitating weight loss. A key aspect of the ketogenic diet is its emphasis on healthy fats and lean proteins. Seniors are encouraged to incorporate foods rich in healthy fats, such as avocados, nuts, seeds, and olive oil, into their diet. These fats provide essential nutrients and promote feelings of fullness and satisfaction, making it easier for seniors to adhere to their dietary goals. Likewise, lean proteins play a crucial role in supporting muscle maintenance and repair. Seniors are encouraged to include sources of lean protein, such as chicken, fish, and tofu, in their meals to ensure adequate protein intake. By preserving muscle mass, the ketogenic diet helps seniors maintain their strength, mobility, and functionality as they age. Beyond physical benefits, achieving and maintaining a healthy weight through the ketogenic diet can have profound effects on seniors' overall well-being. Shedding excess weight, particularly around the abdominal area, reduces the risk of chronic diseases such as diabetes, heart disease, and certain cancers. Additionally, weight loss can boost confidence, improve mood, and enhance quality of life in later years. In essence, weight management and fat loss are vital components of healthy aging for seniors. The ketogenic diet offers a holistic approach to achieving these goals by reducing carbohydrate intake, emphasizing healthy fats and lean proteins, preserving muscle mass, and supporting overall well-being.

2. Improved Metabolic Health

The ketogenic diet has garnered attention for its potential to support brain function and cognitive well-being. By supplying the brain with ketones as an alternative energy source, the ketogenic diet may offer neuroprotective benefits, safeguarding against cognitive decline and neurodegenerative diseases. Numerous studies have indicated that the ketogenic diet holds promise in enhancing memory, cognitive performance, and reducing the risk of neurodegenerative conditions such as Alzheimer's disease and dementia. One essential nutrient abundant in the ketogenic diet, particularly in fatty fish like salmon and mackerel, is docosahexaenoic acid (DHA). DHA is a remarkable omega-3 fatty acid renowned for its role in promoting brain health.

The significance of DHA lies in its ability to preserve the integrity of brain cell membranes. These membranes serve as the guardians of our brain cells, ensuring their structural stability and resilience. DHA acts as a potent protector, fortifying these membranes and shielding them from damage caused by oxidative stress and inflammation. Moreover, DHA facilitates communication between brain cells, fostering the seamless exchange of information within the intricate neural network. By promoting optimal brain function and connectivity, DHA supports various cognitive processes, including learning, memory, and decision-making. In essence, the ketogenic diet offers seniors a holistic approach to enhancing metabolic health and preserving cognitive function. By supplying the brain with ketones and essential nutrients like DHA, the ketogenic diet nourishes and protects the brain, promoting cognitive vitality and reducing the risk of age-related cognitive decline. Embracing the ketogenic lifestyle empowers seniors to prioritize their cognitive well-being and enjoy optimal brain health in their later years.

3. Increased Energy Levels

By relying on fats for fuel, the ketogenic diet provides seniors with sustained and stable energy levels throughout the day, mitigating the fluctuations commonly experienced with carbohydrate-based diets. Many seniors have reported experiencing a significant boost in energy and alertness upon adopting the ketogenic diet. This newfound vitality can have profound implications for daily life, enabling seniors to engage in activities they enjoy with renewed vigor and enthusiasm. The key mechanism behind the ketogenic diet's ability to enhance energy levels lies in its promotion of ketosis, a metabolic state where the body efficiently converts fats into ketones for energy. Ketones serve as a highly efficient and sustainable fuel source, providing the brain and muscles with a steady supply of energy without the need for frequent refueling. Moreover, the ketogenic diet's emphasis on nutrient-dense foods further contributes to improved energy levels in seniors. By prioritizing wholesome fats, lean proteins, and nutrient-rich vegetables, the diet ensures that seniors receive essential vitamins, minerals, and antioxidants necessary for optimal energy production and cellular function. In summary, the ketogenic diet offers seniors a reliable and sustainable solution for maintaining energy levels throughout the day. By harnessing the power of fats as a primary fuel source and prioritizing nutrient-dense foods, the ketogenic diet empowers seniors to enjoy heightened energy, vitality, and well-being as they navigate the challenges of aging.

4. Better Heart Health

The ketogenic diet offers promising benefits in this regard, promoting cardiovascular wellness through various mechanisms. One notable advantage of the ketogenic diet is its ability to regulate lipid profiles, thereby reducing the risk factors associated with cardiovascular disease. By decreasing triglyceride levels and increasing levels of high-density lipoprotein (HDL) cholesterol, the ketogenic diet fosters a heart-healthy environment within the body. Triglycerides are a type of fat found in the bloodstream, and elevated levels are associated with an increased risk of heart disease. The ketogenic diet's emphasis on fat as the primary fuel source leads to a reduction in triglyceride levels, mitigating this risk factor and promoting cardiovascular health. Furthermore, the ketogenic diet has been shown to elevate levels of HDL cholesterol, often referred to as "good" cholesterol.

HDL cholesterol plays a crucial role in removing excess cholesterol from the bloodstream, transporting it to the liver for elimination, and thereby reducing the buildup of plaque in the arteries. By enhancing HDL cholesterol levels, the ketogenic diet further supports heart health and reduces the risk of cardiovascular disease.

5. Appetite Regulation

One of the remarkable aspects of the ketogenic diet is its ability to stabilize blood sugar levels, providing a steady source of energy throughout the day. This stability in blood sugar levels is key to reducing hunger spikes and enhancing appetite control. When you consume carbohydrates in your diet, they can lead to rapid spikes and crashes in blood sugar levels. These fluctuations often result in cravings and overeating, which can be challenging to manage, especially as we age. However, the ketogenic diet takes a different approach. By emphasizing low-carb, high-fat foods, it promotes a consistent and steady blood sugar level. The benefit of this stability is twofold. Firstly, it helps prevent sudden cravings that often derail dietary goals. Secondly, it fosters a feeling of fullness, which can be especially advantageous for older women. This improved appetite control can make it significantly easier to manage food intake and adhere to your dietary objectives.

6. Enhanced Bone Health

Maintaining strong and healthy bones is paramount for seniors, ensuring mobility, independence, and overall well-being as we age. While concerns have been raised regarding the ketogenic diet's impact on bone health, it's possible to adopt a ketogenic eating pattern that supports bone strength and resilience. One essential aspect of promoting bone health on a ketogenic diet is ensuring adequate intake of calcium and vitamin D. These nutrients are critical for bone strength and play a pivotal role in reducing the risk of fractures and osteoporosis in older adults. Leafy green vegetables such as kale and spinach serve as excellent natural sources of calcium, aligning seamlessly with the principles of the ketogenic diet. These nutrient-rich greens can be incorporated into various keto-friendly dishes, providing a substantial boost to your calcium intake and supporting bone health. Furthermore, low-carb dairy products like Greek yogurt and cheese not only supply calcium but also contribute to your vitamin D intake. Vitamin D is essential for calcium absorption and plays a vital role in maintaining optimal bone density and strength. By including these calcium-rich foods in your ketogenic meal plan, you can fortify your bones and ensure they remain strong and resilient throughout the aging process. This is particularly pertinent for seniors, as maintaining bone health is crucial for preserving mobility, preventing fractures, and enhancing overall quality of life in later years.

7. Stable Blood Pressure

The ketogenic diet has shown promise in helping to lower blood pressure in some individuals, which can be particularly beneficial for seniors looking to manage their cardiovascular risk factors. By reducing carbohydrate intake and focusing on healthy fats and lean proteins, the ketogenic diet can have a positive impact on blood pressure levels. Studies have suggested that the diet's ability to promote weight loss, reduce inflammation, and improve insulin sensitivity may contribute to its blood pressure-lowering effects.

By incorporating the ketogenic diet as part of a comprehensive approach to cardiovascular health, seniors can work towards achieving and maintaining stable blood pressure levels, ultimately supporting their overall well-being and quality of life. However, it's important for seniors to monitor their blood pressure regularly, especially if they are taking medications for hypertension. Changes in diet, including adopting a ketogenic approach, may affect medication efficacy and require adjustments under the guidance of a healthcare professional.

8. Mental Health

Emerging research suggests that the ketogenic diet may have potential benefits for mental health, including mood regulation and cognitive function, which are particularly relevant for seniors. The ketogenic diet's emphasis on healthy fats and nutrient-dense foods may play a role in supporting brain health and function. By providing the brain with ketones as an alternative energy source, the diet may offer neuroprotective effects and enhance cognitive function. Moreover, certain nutrients found in foods commonly consumed on a ketogenic diet, such as omega-3 fatty acids and antioxidants, have been associated with improved mood and cognitive performance. These nutrients may help combat inflammation and oxidative stress, which are implicated in age-related cognitive decline and mood disorders. Additionally, the ketogenic diet's potential to stabilize blood sugar levels and improve insulin sensitivity may also contribute to its effects on mental health. Fluctuations in blood sugar levels have been linked to mood swings and cognitive impairment, and by promoting stable blood sugar levels, the diet may help mitigate these effects. While more research is needed to fully understand the relationship between the ketogenic diet and mental health in seniors, preliminary evidence suggests promising avenues for further exploration. By incorporating the ketogenic diet as part of a holistic approach to mental and brain health, seniors can potentially enhance their cognitive function, mood regulation, and overall mental well-being, ultimately supporting a higher quality of life in later years.

9. Reduction of Inflammation

Inflammation is a natural immune response that helps the body fight off harmful invaders and repair damaged tissues. However, chronic inflammation, characterized by persistent activation of the immune system, is linked to various age-related diseases such as heart disease, arthritis, and neurodegenerative disorders. The ketogenic diet has been shown to have anti-inflammatory effects, potentially reducing the risk of these chronic conditions in seniors. The ketogenic diet's anti-inflammatory properties stem from its ability to reduce levels of pro-inflammatory molecules called cytokines while increasing the production of anti-inflammatory compounds. By minimizing chronic inflammation, the ketogenic diet may help alleviate symptoms associated with inflammatory conditions such as joint pain, stiffness, and cognitive decline. Additionally, the ketogenic diet's emphasis on whole, nutrient-dense foods rich in antioxidants further supports its anti-inflammatory effects. Antioxidants help neutralize harmful free radicals, which are molecules that can cause oxidative damage and contribute to inflammation. By incorporating antioxidant-rich foods like berries, leafy greens, and nuts, seniors can enhance the anti-inflammatory benefits of the ketogenic diet and promote overall health and well-being.

In summary, the ketogenic diet's ability to reduce chronic inflammation may offer significant benefits to seniors by lowering the risk of age-related diseases and improving overall quality of life.

10. Improved Diabetes Management

Type 2 diabetes is a prevalent chronic condition among seniors, characterized by high blood sugar levels and insulin resistance. The ketogenic diet's low-carbohydrate, moderate-protein, and high-fat composition may offer advantages in managing type 2 diabetes by improving insulin sensitivity and glycemic control. When carbohydrates are restricted, as in the ketogenic diet, blood sugar levels remain stable, reducing the need for insulin secretion. This can help prevent spikes in blood sugar levels after meals and promote more consistent energy levels throughout the day. Additionally, the ketogenic diet encourages the body to utilize fat for fuel instead of glucose, which can lead to weight loss and reduced fat accumulation in tissues like the liver and pancreas, improving insulin sensitivity over time. Several studies have demonstrated the efficacy of the ketogenic diet in improving glycemic control and reducing medication dependence in individuals with type 2 diabetes. By adopting a ketogenic diet under the guidance of a healthcare professional, seniors with diabetes may experience better blood sugar management, reduced risk of diabetes-related complications, and improved overall health outcomes. In conclusion, the ketogenic diet offers promise in improving diabetes management for seniors by enhancing insulin sensitivity, stabilizing blood sugar levels, and promoting weight loss.

11. Better Sleep Quality

Quality sleep is essential for overall health and well-being, yet many seniors struggle with sleep-related issues such as insomnia, sleep fragmentation, and sleep apnea. The ketogenic diet may offer benefits in improving sleep quality and duration, thereby enhancing seniors' overall sleep experience. One mechanism through which the ketogenic diet may improve sleep quality is by promoting the production of neurotransmitters and hormones that regulate sleep-wake cycles. For example, the ketogenic diet has been shown to increase levels of gamma-aminobutyric acid (GABA), a neurotransmitter that promotes relaxation and sleep. Additionally, ketones produced during ketosis may exert a calming effect on the brain, leading to deeper and more restorative sleep. Furthermore, the ketogenic diet's ability to stabilize blood sugar levels may help prevent nighttime awakenings caused by fluctuations in blood glucose. By reducing carbohydrate intake and minimizing insulin spikes, the ketogenic diet can promote more stable energy levels throughout the night, allowing seniors to enjoy uninterrupted sleep. In summary, the ketogenic diet may offer seniors a natural and effective approach to improving sleep quality, enhancing overall health, and promoting a greater sense of well-being.

12. Increased Self-Esteem and Psychological Well-being

Weight loss and improvements in overall health can have profound effects on self-esteem and psychological well-being in seniors. Adopting a ketogenic diet that promotes sustainable weight loss and health improvement may contribute to enhanced self-esteem, mood, and quality of life.

As seniors experience positive changes in their physical health, such as weight loss, increased energy levels, and improved mobility, they may also experience a boost in self-confidence and self-esteem. Achieving personal health goals through dietary changes can instill a sense of accomplishment and empowerment, fostering a positive self-image and greater self-worth. Additionally, improvements in physical health often translate to improvements in mental health and psychological well-being. Seniors may experience reduced feelings of anxiety and depression, increased vitality and zest for life, and greater overall life satisfaction as a result of adopting a ketogenic diet and achieving their health-related goals. In conclusion, the ketogenic diet offers seniors an opportunity to improve their physical health and well-being, which can have far-reaching effects on self-esteem, mood, and overall quality of life.

3.2 Side Effects of the Ketogenic Diet for Seniors

As we explore the ketogenic diet and its potential benefits for seniors, it's essential to also acknowledge and address potential risks and challenges associated with this dietary approach. While the keto diet offers many advantages, it's crucial to make informed choices and be aware of possible difficulties that may arise during your journey.

1. Nutrient Intake. One challenge of the ketogenic diet is ensuring that you receive an adequate intake of vital nutrients. The diet restricts carbohydrates, which are a primary source of many vitamins and minerals. To mitigate this risk, it's essential to focus on a well-balanced keto diet that incorporates a variety of non-starchy vegetables, lean proteins, and healthy fats. Additionally, consider taking supplements to cover any potential nutrient gaps, especially important for seniors who may have specific nutritional needs.

2. Digestive Issues. Some individuals may experience digestive discomfort when transitioning to a keto diet, including constipation, diarrhea, or other gastrointestinal disturbances. To address these challenges, it's advisable to gradually increase fiber intake from keto-friendly sources like leafy greens, nuts, and seeds. Staying hydrated and incorporating fermented foods can also promote digestive health.

3. Potential Side Effects. The keto diet can sometimes lead to side effects known as the "keto flu," which may include fatigue, headache, and nausea during the initial stages of ketosis. While these symptoms are typically temporary, it's vital to stay well-hydrated, consume adequate electrolytes, and get plenty of rest to ease the transition.

4. Monitoring Ketosis. Achieving and maintaining ketosis, the metabolic state where your body burns fat for fuel, is a primary goal of the ketogenic diet. However, it can be challenging to monitor your ketone levels accurately. Consider using ketone testing strips or blood ketone meters to track your progress and ensure you are in a state of ketosis.

5. Individual Variability. Keep in mind that individual responses to the ketogenic diet can vary. What works well for one person might not have the same effect on another. Therefore, it's vital to listen to your body, pay attention to how you feel, and make adjustments to your dietary plan as needed.

6. Medical Considerations. Some medications may interact with the ketogenic diet and have different effects. It's vital to consult with a healthcare provider to monitor medication effectiveness and make any necessary adjustments while following the diet. Certain medical conditions may require modified versions of the diet or close monitoring.

7. Bone Health. Seniors may be more susceptible to bone health issues like osteoporosis. The ketogenic diet can potentially affect calcium and magnesium levels in the body. It's important to ensure you're getting an adequate amount of these nutrients through foods or supplements if necessary to support bone health.

8. Dehydration. The ketogenic diet can have a diuretic effect, meaning it may increase fluid loss through urine. Seniors may already be more susceptible to dehydration, so it's crucial to maintain proper hydration levels while on the diet. To prevent dehydration while following the ketogenic diet, it's vital to have a clear understanding of your daily water intake needs. Incorporate regular water intake into your daily routine and be attentive to your body's signals for thirst.

9. Long-Term Sustainability. Maintaining a ketogenic diet over the long term can be challenging for some individuals. Seniors should consider the sustainability of the diet and whether it aligns with their lifestyle and preferences.

3.3 Managing Ketogenic Diet Side Effects

As seniors embark on their ketogenic journey, it's essential to tailor the diet to meet their unique needs and address potential challenges they may encounter along the way. One key consideration is the potential impact of age-related changes on nutrient requirements and metabolic processes. Seniors may have different nutritional needs compared to younger individuals, necessitating adjustments to ensure they receive adequate nutrients while following the ketogenic diet. Additionally, seniors may face challenges such as decreased appetite, dental issues, or difficulty swallowing, which can affect their ability to adhere to the diet. It's crucial to take these factors into account and find creative solutions to overcome barriers to dietary compliance. This may involve modifying food textures or meal frequencies to accommodate individual preferences and physical limitations. Furthermore, managing potential side effects of the ketogenic diet is essential for seniors to ensure a smooth transition into ketosis and optimize their experience. Here are some tips for managing potential side effects:

✓ A few individuals may experience flu-like symptoms when initially transitioning into ketosis. Combat this by staying hydrated, replenishing electrolytes, and ensuring adequate rest.

✓ A few individuals may experience constipation on a ketogenic diet. Increase your fiber intake through low-carb vegetables and consider adding a fiber supplement if needed.

✓ Muscle cramps can result from electrolyte imbalances. Include magnesium-rich foods or supplements to help prevent cramping.

✓ Ketosis may lead to increased fluid loss through urine. Drink water consistently to stay hydrated, and consider adding an electrolyte supplement if needed.

- ✓ A few individuals may experience increased hunger or cravings initially. Focus on satisfying, keto-friendly foods and practice mindful eating to manage these urges.

- ✓ While your body adapts to ketosis, you might notice changes in energy levels. Ensure you're consuming enough calories and give your body time to adjust.

- ✓ Be mindful of potential nutrient deficiencies, especially calcium and potassium. Consult with a healthcare provider to determine if supplementation is necessary.

- ✓ Monitor your cholesterol levels regularly, as a ketogenic diet can affect cholesterol markers. Consult with your healthcare provider to assess and manage any changes.

- ✓ Navigating social gatherings and dining out can be challenging. Plan ahead, communicate your dietary preferences, and be prepared with keto-friendly options to stay on track.

3.4 Embracing the Ketogenic Lifestyle for Seniors

Embracing the ketogenic lifestyle as a senior, particularly for those in their golden years, can offer a transformative and fulfilling journey. It's essential to approach this lifestyle change with confidence and enthusiasm. Here's a heartfelt guide crafted to inspire and support you on your ketogenic voyage:

- ✓ **Believe in Your Resilience:** Age is merely a number, and within you lies the strength and resilience to enact positive changes in your life. Embrace the notion that prioritizing your health and well-being is a timeless endeavor.

- ✓ **Begin Gradually:** Ease into your ketogenic journey with small, incremental adjustments to your diet. Allow your body the time it needs to adapt to this new way of eating. Progress at a pace that feels comfortable, focusing on sustainability rather than rapid changes.

- ✓ **Seek Support and Expert Advice**

- ✓ **Diversify Your Meals:** Keep your ketogenic adventure vibrant and enticing by exploring an array of keto-friendly recipes and ingredients. Don't hesitate to experiment with diverse flavors and textures. Variety not only adds excitement to your culinary experiences but also ensures a well-rounded nutritional intake.

- ✓ **Take Pleasure in Cooking:** Cooking can be an enjoyable and creative pursuit. Embrace the joy of preparing keto-friendly meals by experimenting with new recipes and innovative cooking techniques. Finding delight in the culinary process can make the ketogenic lifestyle an enriching part of your daily routine.

- ✓ **Educate Yourself:** Knowledge empowers. Take the initiative to learn about the ketogenic lifestyle, its fundamental principles, and the potential benefits it offers. Understanding the underlying rationale behind this dietary approach can reinforce your commitment and resolve.

- ✓ **Celebrate Milestones**

✓ **Cultivate a Positive Mindset:** Foster a compassionate and optimistic outlook towards yourself and your journey. Practice patience and self-understanding, recognizing that each step forward is a stride towards enhanced health and vitality.

✓ **Nurture a Healthy Relationship with Food:** Develop a positive and balanced relationship with food. Understand that the ketogenic lifestyle is not about deprivation but rather about nourishing your body with wholesome, gratifying foods. By maintaining a favorable attitude towards food, you can sustain this dietary approach in the long term.

✓ **Remain Curious:** Maintain a spirit of curiosity and openness to new experiences and knowledge. The ketogenic journey presents an opportunity for personal growth and exploration.

✓ **Enjoy the Ride:** Ultimately, remember that your ketogenic journey is not solely about reaching a destination; it's about relishing the journey itself. Treasure each moment, indulge in delicious meals, and revel in the revitalization it brings to your life.

Embracing the ketogenic lifestyle as a senior marks a significant stride towards enhanced health and well-being. Approach it with determination, self-compassion, and a spirit of adventure. Your journey is uniquely yours, and each day presents an opportunity to thrive on the path to wellness.

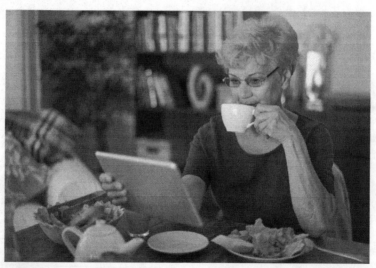

Challenges and Solutions

Now, let's explore some tips for overcoming the challenges that may arise while following the ketogenic diet.

1. Food Choices at Social Gatherings. Maintaining a ketogenic diet can be particularly challenging when attending social gatherings where high-carb options abound. However, with some strategic planning, it's possible to stick to your dietary goals even in these situations. Here are some practical tips:

✓ **Lean Proteins:** Look for dishes featuring lean proteins such as grilled chicken, turkey, or fish. These options are typically low in carbohydrates and can serve as the cornerstone of your meal.

✓ **Vegetables:** Load up on non-starchy vegetables like leafy greens, broccoli, cauliflower, and asparagus. These vegetables provide essential nutrients and fiber without significantly impacting your carb intake.

✓ **Healthy Fats:** Seek out sources of healthy fats like avocados, olive oil, and nuts. These fats not only help you feel satiated but also provide crucial nutrients for overall health.

✓ **Avoid Sugary Sauces:** Exercise caution with sauces and dressings, as they often contain hidden sugars and carbohydrates. Opt for options with minimal sugar content or request sauces on the side to control your intake.

2. Effective Communication. Maintaining effective communication is key to enjoying social events while adhering to your ketogenic diet:

✓ **Express Your Preferences:** Be open and upfront about your dietary preferences and restrictions with hosts or friends. Most people are understanding and will appreciate your honesty, making it easier to accommodate your needs.

✓ **Offer to Contribute:** When attending potluck-style gatherings, offer to bring a dish that aligns with your keto diet. Not only does this ensure you have a suitable option to enjoy, but it also introduces others to delicious keto-friendly recipes.

✓ **Ask Questions:** If you're unsure about the ingredients used in a dish, don't hesitate to ask the host for clarification. Being informed about what you're eating helps you make informed choices that align with your dietary goals.

✓ **Special Requests:** Don't shy away from making special requests when dining out. Many restaurants are willing to accommodate dietary needs, so don't hesitate to ask for modifications to suit your keto lifestyle.

3. Strategic Meal Planning. Planning ahead is a valuable strategy for staying committed to your ketogenic diet during social gatherings:

✓ **Plan Your Dish:** If possible, collaborate with the host to plan a keto-friendly dish that suits your dietary needs. This ensures you have a satisfying option available that aligns with your goal

✓ **Prepare in Advance:** Consider preparing keto-friendly snacks or appetizers ahead of time, ensuring you always have something suitable to munch on during the event.

✓ **Bring Your Own (BYO):** If necessary, bring your own keto-friendly dish to social gatherings. This guarantees you'll have a meal option available that meets your dietary requirements.

✓ **Eat Beforehand:** If you anticipate limited keto options at the event, consider eating a small keto-friendly meal or snack beforehand. This helps curb your appetite and reduces the temptation to indulge in non-keto foods.

4. Managing Cravings. Understanding the difference between genuine hunger and cravings is crucial. True hunger is characterized by distinct physical sensations and signals from your body, including:

✓ **Stomach Sensations:** True hunger often manifests as a sensation of emptiness or a gentle rumbling in the stomach. This physical signal indicates that your body needs nourishment.

✓ **Physical Weakness:** Genuine hunger can lead to feelings of weakness or low energy levels. Your body signals the need for fuel to regain vitality.

✓ **Consistent Timing:** True hunger tends to follow a consistent schedule, aligning with your typical meal times. It builds gradually and becomes more noticeable as time since your last meal or snack increases.

✓ **Lack of Food Obsession:** When you're genuinely hungry, you may think about food in a practical, non-obsessive way. The thought of eating is driven by a physical need rather than an emotional craving.

In addition to understanding hunger cues, it's helpful to have practical strategies for managing food temptations:

✓ **Distraction:** When experiencing cravings unrelated to genuine hunger, try engaging in enjoyable or relaxing activities to divert your attention away from food.

✓ **Stay Hydrated:** Drinking a glass of water can help reduce feelings of hunger and provide a temporary sense of fullness.

✓ **Employ Stress Management Techniques:** Food is often used as a means to cope with emotional stress. Learning stress management techniques such as meditation, deep breathing, or yoga can help reduce reliance on food as a coping mechanism.

Having keto-friendly snacks readily available is vital when cravings strike. Here's a detailed look at handling snacking:

✓ **Nuts:** Almonds, walnuts, and macadamia nuts are excellent choices for healthy fats and a satisfying crunch.

✓ **Seeds:** Chia seeds, flaxseeds, and pumpkin seeds provide fiber and nutrients.

✓ **Cheese:** Cheese sticks or cubes are rich in both flavor and healthy fats.

✓ **Vegetables with Dip:** Crisp, low-carb vegetables like cucumber, celery, and bell peppers paired with keto-friendly dips.

Of course, portion control matters when snacking. Properly portioned snacks serve several purposes, including:

✓ **Managing Calorie Intake:** By controlling the quantity of snacks you consume, you can better manage your overall calorie intake. This is vital for weight management and staying in a calorie deficit if your goal is weight loss.

✓ **Staying within Daily Carb Limits:** For a ketogenic diet, it's vital to monitor your carbohydrate intake closely. Proper portion control ensures that you don't exceed your daily carb limit while enjoying snacks.

- ✓ **Curbing Cravings:** Snacking in moderation can help curb cravings without derailing your diet. By eating the right portion size, you satisfy your hunger without overindulging.

Here there are some practical strategies for effective portion control when snacking:

- ✓ **Measuring Portions:** Using measuring teacups or a food scale to measure out your snacks can be an eye-opening experience. It helps you become aware of what an appropriate portion looks like.

- ✓ **Pre-Portioning:** Pre-portioning snacks into individual servings can prevent mindless eating. It's especially helpful for snacks like nuts or seeds, where it's easy to lose track of how much you've eaten.

- ✓ **Snack Packaging:** Choosing snacks that come in single-presenting packages can simplify portion control. This eliminates the need for measuring and helps you avoid overindulging.

Paying attention to these physical signals can help you make mindful choices and respond to your body's actual nutritional needs. Emotions often lead to cravings, which can mimic feelings of hunger. Recognizing emotional triggers is vital to differentiate between emotional desires and genuine hunger. Common emotional triggers include:

- ✓ **Stress:** Stress can create a desire for comforting foods as a way to cope with emotional tension. This can lead to cravings for specific comfort foods.

- ✓ **Boredom:** When you're bored, food can become a source of entertainment or distraction. This may lead to cravings even when you're not truly hungry.

- ✓ **Sadness or Loneliness:** Emotional states like sadness or loneliness can trigger cravings for foods that provide a temporary sense of comfort or pleasure.

- ✓ **Habitual Eating:** A fewtimes, you may feel like eating simply out of habit, not because you're hungry. These habitual eating patterns can lead to cravings that are not based on genuine hunger.

By practicing mindful eating, you can enhance your ability to differentiate between true hunger and cravings. Mindful eating is a practice that can help you differentiate between genuine hunger and cravings. It involves:

- ✓ **Paying Attention:** Being fully present during meals and snacks, focusing on the sensory experience of eating, including taste, texture, and aroma.

- ✓ **Engage Your Senses:** Pay attention to the colors, smells, and textures of your food. It enhances the experience.

- ✓ **Chew Thoroughly:** Chew your food slowly and thoroughly. It allows your body to signal when it's full.

- ✓ **Pause Between Bites:** Put your utensils down between bites. This slows the pace of your meal.

- ✓ **Appreciate Your Food:** Be grateful for the nourishment your meal provides.

- ✓ **Listening to Your Body:** Tuning into your body's hunger and fullness cues. Before eating, ask yourself if you're truly hungry, and after eating, assess your level of fullness.

- ✓ **Eating with Awareness:** Avoiding distractions while eating, like watching TV or scrolling through your phone. This allows you to savor each bite and be more in tune with your body's signals.

- ✓ **Non-Judgmental Observation:** Approaching your eating habits with curiosity and without self-criticism. Mindful eating is about developing a compassionate and non-judgmental relationship with food.

- ✓ **Savoring Each Bite**: As we age, our sense of taste can change. Mindful eating encourages savoring each bite, making meals more enjoyable.

- ✓ **Portion Control:** Mindful eating helps with portion control, preventing overeating, which is vital when following a ketogenic diet.

- ✓ **Beverage Choices:** Choose water, unsweetened tea, or sparkling water as your beverages to avoid unnecessary sugar and carbs from sodas and sugary drinks.

5. Customized Sleep Strategies. Ensuring adequate sleep is crucial, especially when following a ketogenic diet regimen. Quality sleep supports various metabolic processes and overall well-being, making customized sleep strategies essential for success on a ketogenic journey.

- ✓ **Sleep Environment:** Creating a comfortable sleep environment is vital. This includes optimizing factors like lighting, noise, and temperature in your bedroom to promote relaxation and restful sleep.

- ✓ **Sleep Hygiene:** Establishing good sleep hygiene practices is key. This involves maintaining a regular sleep schedule and developing a bedtime routine that supports restorative sleep

- ✓ **Nutrition and Timing:** Your dietary choices and meal timing can significantly impact sleep quality. Adjusting your eating patterns to avoid heavy meals close to bedtime and incorporating sleep-promoting nutrients can improve sleep.

- ✓ **Relaxation Techniques:** Implementing relaxation techniques such as deep breathing or gentle yoga before bedtime can help calm the mind and body, enhancing your ability to fall asleep and stay asleep.

6. Occasional Treats. How to incorporate occasional treats into your ketogenic lifestyle without compromising your progress? Making informed choices when selecting treats is crucial. You can opt for dark chocolate with a higher cocoa content as it tends to be lower in carbohydrates compared to milk chocolate. Additionally, consider sugar-free or keto-friendly desserts as suitable alternatives to traditional high-carb treats. As I have already said before, practicing moderation is key to mindful indulgence. On a ketogenic diet, you have a specific daily limit for carbohydrate consumption to maintain ketosis. Consuming too many carbs, even from keto-friendly sources, can potentially disrupt ketosis and hinder your progress. Be mindful of how the occasional treat fits into your daily carb budget.

Moreover, it's vital to find a balance between enjoying occasional treats and staying true to your keto goals. Remember that these treats should enhance your overall keto experience rather than become the primary focus of your diet. They are a part of a sustainable approach to keto, allowing you to savor special moments without compromising your long-term health objectives. By practicing moderation and staying within your daily carb limits, you can relish occasional treats while ensuring that your ketogenic journey remains on track. This balanced approach not only supports your dietary success but also promotes a healthier relationship with food and helps you achieve and maintain your desired health outcomes.

3.5 Addressing Common Queries and Concerns

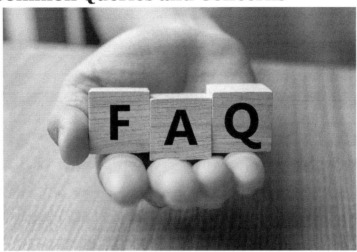

As you journey through the pages of "Keto Diet For Seniors," you may encounter recurring questions that warrant revisiting. Repetition reinforces understanding, ensuring that essential concepts are not only absorbed but also ingrained.

1. Is the Ketogenic Diet Safe for Seniors?

The ketogenic diet can be safe and beneficial for seniors, but it requires awareness and caution. Before embarking on any new dietary regimen, especially if you have underlying health issues or take medications, consult with a healthcare provider. Personalizing the diet to align with your unique health needs is crucial.

2. Is Ketosis Safe for Seniors?

While ketosis is generally safe for seniors, individual responses may vary. Ketosis, a metabolic state where the body burns fat for fuel instead of carbohydrates, can offer stable energy levels. However, it's essential to monitor ketone levels, especially when initiating the diet. Seek personalized guidance from a healthcare provider.

3. How Can I Maintain Hydration on the Keto Diet?

The ketogenic diet can increase fluid loss through urine, potentially leading to dehydration, particularly in older adults. Ensure proper hydration by consuming approximately 8 to 10 cups (64 to 80 oz.) of water daily, adjusting based on individual needs. Pay attention to thirst signals and prioritize adequate hydration.

4. Is the Keto Diet Sustainable for Seniors in the Long Term?

The sustainability of the ketogenic diet varies among individuals. To enhance sustainability, incorporate diverse keto-friendly recipes and meal components to add variety. Embrace the pleasure of keto cooking, experimenting with flavors and textures. Remember, sustainability extends beyond the diet to encompass enjoying the lifestyle journey.

5. How Can I Manage Appetite on the Ketogenic Diet?

The ketogenic diet can aid in stabilizing blood sugar levels, reducing hunger spikes, and improving appetite control, particularly for older adults. Consuming low-carb, high-fat foods promotes stable blood sugar, preventing sudden cravings and promoting satiety. Enhanced appetite control facilitates managing food intake and adhering to dietary goals.

6. Can I Meet Nutritional Needs on the Keto Diet?

A well-balanced ketogenic diet can supply essential nutrients. Ensure adequate intake of vitamins and minerals by incorporating a variety of non-starchy vegetables, lean proteins, and healthy fats. Consider supplements to address potential nutrient gaps, especially for seniors with specific nutritional requirements.

7. Can I Enjoy Social Gatherings and Dining Out on Keto?

Navigating social gatherings and dining out while following the ketogenic diet is feasible with proper planning. Communicate dietary preferences to hosts or restaurants in advance. Prepare with keto-friendly options and focus on the social aspect rather than feeling restricted by dietary choices.

8. How Can Seniors Prevent the "Keto Flu"?

The "keto flu," characterized by symptoms like fatigue and nausea during the transition into ketosis, can be prevented or alleviated by prioritizing hydration, replenishing electrolytes, and ensuring ample rest during the initial stages of ketosis.

9. What Role Does the Ketogenic Diet Play in Promoting Healthy Aging and Longevity?

The ketogenic diet may contribute to healthy aging and longevity by regulating blood sugar levels, reducing inflammation, and supporting cognitive function. By promoting fat utilization as the primary energy source, the diet may aid in weight management and mitigate the risk of age-related ailments.

10. Are There Keto-Friendly Foods That Enhance Joint Health for Seniors?

Certain keto-friendly foods, such as fatty fish rich in omega-3 fatty acids, can benefit joint health by possessing anti-inflammatory properties. Additionally, incorporating leafy greens and nuts can provide essential vitamins and minerals that support joint health.

11. Can the Ketogenic Diet Assist in Managing Age-Related Conditions Like Osteoporosis?

The ketogenic diet can support bone health by providing calcium and vitamin D through foods like leafy greens and dairy products.

By reducing sugar and processed food consumption, the diet may also aid in preventing bone loss.

12. What Are the Social and Emotional Benefits of the Ketogenic Diet for Seniors?

Beyond physical health, the ketogenic diet can foster social connections and emotional well-being. Sharing dietary experiences can cultivate a sense of community, while the diet's impact on blood sugar stability may enhance mood and energy levels.

13. How Does the Ketogenic Diet Affect Weight Loss for Seniors?

The ketogenic diet can facilitate weight loss in seniors by promoting fat burning through reduced carbohydrate intake and increased healthy fats consumption.

14. What Are Some Common Challenges Seniors May Face on a Keto Diet?

Seniors may encounter challenges such as adapting to a low-carb diet, maintaining electrolyte balance, and managing potential side effects like the "keto flu." Awareness of these challenges is crucial, and seeking guidance when needed is recommended.

15. Can the Ketogenic Diet Help Manage Age-Related Health Conditions?

Preliminary studies suggest potential benefits of the ketogenic diet for age-related conditions like cognitive decline and metabolic health. However, cautious consideration and medical advice are essential when considering dietary changes.

16. Are There Keto-Friendly Foods That Support Bone Health in Seniors?

Certain keto-friendly foods, including leafy greens, dairy products, and fatty fish, provide essential nutrients for bone health, contributing to seniors' overall bone density support.

17. How Does the Ketogenic Diet Impact Energy Levels and Vitality in Seniors?

The ketogenic diet may offer seniors a stable energy source by utilizing fat as the primary fuel. Some seniors report improved vitality and mental clarity, although individual responses may vary.

18. What Are the Key Benefits of the Keto Diet for Seniors?

The ketogenic diet presents benefits such as weight management, improved metabolic health, and enhanced mental clarity, particularly beneficial for seniors aiming to maintain vitality and manage weight.

19. Is the Keto Diet Suitable for Seniors With Medical Conditions?

While adaptable to address specific health needs, seniors with medical conditions should consult healthcare professionals for personalized guidance to ensure safety and effectiveness.

20. What Are the Risks and Side Effects of the Keto Diet for Older Adults?

Potential side effects of the keto diet, including the "keto flu," digestive issues, and medication interactions, should be carefully considered by seniors. Consulting healthcare providers is crucial to mitigate risks effectively.

21. How Can Seniors Transition to the Keto Diet Safely?

Seniors should transition to the keto diet gradually, monitor their health closely, and seek guidance from healthcare providers. Gradually reducing carbohydrate intake while increasing healthy fats facilitates a safe and smooth transition.

3.6 Real-Life Transformations on the Ketogenic Diet

Within the pages of this book, I have the privilege of sharing with you a compilation of inspiring success stories that showcase the transformative power of the ketogenic diet for both men and women over 60 and 70. While the stories featured here are just a glimpse into the thousands of success stories that exist, they hold the power to inspire and illuminate the possibilities that lie ahead. You probably know that I am Melinda Francis, a nutritionist, and the women whose journeys you will read about are not only my patients, but they are also individuals who have generously chosen to share their personal experiences. These stories offer a glimpse into the real-life impact of keto diet on the lives of seniors, showcasing the resilience, determination, and vitality that can be achieved through this approach. As you read through these narratives, I hope you find inspiration and insights that resonate with your own journey toward improved health and well-being. Each story is a testament to the potential for positive change, and it is our sincere hope that they empower you to embrace the possibilities that the keto diet can bring to your life.

John's Journey to Vibrant Health. John, a vibrant 75-year-old, embarked on his ketogenic journey to address weight management issues and low energy levels. Through dedication to the ketogenic lifestyle, Johnexperienced gradual weight loss and newfound energy, demonstrating that age is not a barrier to achieving remarkable health improvements.

Susan's Cognitive Enhancements. At 72, Susan was concerned about her cognitive health and occasional memory lapses. By adopting the ketogenic diet, Susan noticed significant improvements in her memory and cognitive performance, highlighting the potential neuroprotective benefits of this dietary approach for seniors.

Peter's Active Lifestyle. Determined to lead an active life at 62, Peter discovered that the ketogenic diet provided sustained energy levels, enabling him to enjoy daily activities such as walks, yoga, and gardening. His increased vitality and reduced hunger spikes made maintaining an active lifestyle more achievable than ever.

Eleanor's Heart Health Journey. Eleanor, aged 78, turned to the ketogenic diet to address concerns about her heart health. With guidance, she successfully achieved her goal of lowering triglyceride levels and enhancing overall cardiovascular well-being, showcasing the potential benefits of the ketogenic diet for heart health in seniors.

Linda's Weight Management Success. Struggling with weight management for years, Linda, at 71, found success through the appetite-regulating effects of the ketogenic diet. By controlling cravings and reducing overeating, Linda achieved her weight loss goals while enjoying satisfying and nutritious meals.

Evelyn's Journey to Mental Clarity. Meet Evelyn, a 68-year-old woman who struggled with mental fog and lack of mental clarity. She decided to try the ketogenic diet as a potential solution. After transitioning to a low-carb, high-fat diet, Evelyn noticed a significant improvement in her cognitive abilities. She felt more focutilized and mentally sharp, allowing her to engage in activities she had once found challenging.

Adam's Journey to Freedom from Medications. At 74, Adam battled mental fog and lack of clarity before turning to the ketogenic diet. Transitioning to a low-carb, high-fat diet brought significant improvements in cognitive abilities, allowing Adam to engage in activities with renewed focus and mental sharpness.

Dorothy's Vibrant Golden Years. Dorothy, at 80, embraced the ketogenic diet to enhance her energy levels and vitality. With family support, she engaged in daily activities like dancing and volunteering, serving as an inspiration for seniors looking to lead active and fulfilling lives.

Ruth's Resilience and Weight Loss. Facing health challenges at 75, including weight management issues, Ruth found resilience through the ketogenic diet. Her commitment led to weight loss and increased confidence in her daily life, highlighting the transformative effects of the ketogenic diet on physical and emotional well-being.

Andrew's Journey to Healthy Aging. At 70, Andrew embarked on a ketogenic journey to embrace healthy aging. Integrating keto-friendly foods, he found his way to improved bone health and overall vitality, showcasing the diet's potential to support the specific health needs of older adults.

These real-life success stories illustrate how the ketogenic diet can empower men and women over 60 and 70 to lead vibrant, fulfilling lives. Each journey underscores the positive impact of the ketogenic diet on various aspects of health and well-being, transcending age barriers and offering hope for a healthier future.

Chapter 4: KETO GROCERY LIST

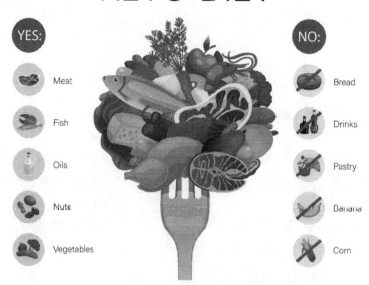

4.1 Essential Foods for Your Ketogenic Journey

As you embark on your ketogenic journey as a senior, it's crucial to stock your kitchen with the right foods to support your new dietary lifestyle. In this section, we'll explore the essential foods seniors should consider adding to their grocery list when following the ketogenic diet.

1. Healthy Fats

✓ Avocados

✓ Coconut oil

✓ Olive oil

✓ Grass-fed butter

Healthy fats are the cornerstone of the ketogenic diet. These fats provide vital nutrients and are a primary source of energy on keto.

2. Protein Sources

✓ Skinless poultry (chicken, turkey)

✓ Lean cuts of beef or pork

✓ Fatty fish (salmon, mackerel)

✓ Eggs (organic and pasture-raised)

Lean proteins are vital for muscle maintenance and overall health. Opt for organic and pasture-raised options when possible.

3. Low-Carb Vegetables

✓ Leafy greens (spinach, kale, arugula)

✓ Broccoli

✓ Cauliflower

✓ Zucchini

✓ Asparagus

✓ Bell peppers

✓ Cucumbers

Non-starchy vegetables are rich in vitamins, minerals, and fiber while being low in carbs. These vegetables are versatile and can be utilized in various keto-friendly recipes.

4. Nuts and Seeds

✓ Almonds   ✓ Chia seeds

✓ Walnuts   ✓ Flaxseeds

Nuts and seeds are excellent sources of healthy fats and provide a satisfying crunch.

5. Dairy Products

✓ Cheese (various types like cheddar, mozzarella, and cream cheese)

✓ Full-fat yogurt (unsweetened)

✓ Heavy cream

If you tolerate dairy, include these items. These dairy products can include flavor and richness to your keto meals.

6. Berries

✓ Strawberries   ✓ Raspberries

✓ Blueberries

While fruits are generally limited on keto due to their sugar content, berries are lower in carbs and can be enjoyed in moderation.

7. Herbs and Spices

✓ Garlic   ✓ Oregano

✓ Basil   ✓ Cinnamon

Enhance the flavor of your meals with herbs and spices. They will include depth and variety to your dishes.

8. Keto-Friendly Sweeteners

✓ Stevia   ✓ Monk fruit sweetener

✓ Erythritol

If you have a sweet tooth, look for keto-friendly sweeteners. These can be utilized as sugar substitutes in keto-friendly desserts.

9. Canned and Jarred Items

✓ Canned tuna or salmon   ✓ Pickles

✓ Olives

These canned and jarred products are keto-friendly. Check labels for added sugars and choose options with no or minimal carbs.

10. Keto-Friendly Snacks

✓ Pork rinds   ✓ Beef jerky

✓   Sugar-free dark chocolate

Keep keto snacks on hand for when cravings strike. These snacks can help you stay on track while satisfying your munchies.

11. Keto-Friendly Drinks

✓   **Water:** Water is vital for maintaining hydration and overall health. It's the best choice for a keto-friendly beverage.

✓   **Unsweetened Tea:** Teas like green tea, black tea, and herbal tea are excellent options. Make sure not to include sugar or high-carb sweeteners.

✓   **Black Coffee:** Black coffee is a low-calorie and low-carb beverage, but avoid adding sugar. You can include cream or butter if you follow a variant of the ketogenic diet known as "bulletproof coffee."

✓   **Natural Sparkling Water:** Sugar-free sparkling water is a refreshing and keto-friendly choice.

✓   **Bone Broth:** Bone broth is rich in nutrients and can be an excellent beverage to support hydration and electrolyte balance during a ketogenic diet.

✓   **Erythritol or Stevia-Based Drinks:** A few beverages sweetened with erythritol or stevia can be keto-friendly options. Just check the labels to ensure they don't contain high-carb components.

✓   **Coconut Water (in moderation):** While coconut water contains some carbohydrates, it can be consumed in moderation if it fits within your daily carb limit. It's a natural source of electrolytes.

✓   **Keto Smoothies (homemade):** You can make keto-friendly smoothies using components like unsweetened almond milk, low-carb berries, spinach, and a keto-friendly sweetener like stevia or erythritol.

Remember to read labels and check for hidden sugars or high-carb additives in any packaged drinks.

4.2 Supplements

Depending on your specific dietary needs, you may consider adding supplements like electrolytes or vitamins to support your health. Consult with a healthcare professional for personalized recommendations.

✓   **Multivitamin and Mineral Supplement:** To ensure you meet your daily nutrient needs.

✓   **Vitamin D:** Especially important for older adults to support bone health and overall wellbeing.

✓   **Omega-3 Fatty Acids:** Fish oil supplements can help with joint health and inflammation.

✓   **Electrolyte Supplements:** Potassium, magnesium, and sodium supplements can help maintain electrolyte balance on a ketogenic diet.

✓   **Collagen Powder:** Supports skin, hair, and joint health.

✓ **Fiber Supplement (if needed):** Psyllium husk or other keto-friendly fiber supplements to support digestive health.

✓ **Calcium and Magnesium:** Calcium is important for bone health, especially in older women, while magnesium supports heart and muscle health.

✓ **Vitamin B12:** Older adults may have an increased need for vitamin B12, which is vital for nerve and cognitive health.

✓ **Probiotics:** Probiotics can help support digestive and immune health.

✓ **Coenzyme Q10 (CoQ10):** This antioxidant may help support heart health and energy production.

4.3 Foods To Avoid

1. Sugar

- ✗ White sugar
- ✗ Brown sugar
- ✗ Honey
- ✗ Maple syrup
- ✗ Agave nectar

Avoid all forms of sugar.

2. Grains

- ✗ Wheat
- ✗ Rice
- ✗ Oats
- ✗ Corn

Eliminate grains, as they are high in carbohydrates.

3. Starchy Vegetables

- ✗ Potatoes
- ✗ Sweet potatoes
- ✗ Peas

Limit starchy vegetables, as they contain more carbs.

4. Processed Foods

- ✗ Chips
- ✗ Cookies
- ✗ Sugary snacks

5. High-Carb Fruits

- ✗ Bananas
- ✗ Grapes
- ✗ Mangoes

6. Legumes

- ✗ Beans
- ✗ Lentils
- ✗ Chickpeas

7. Low-Fat Dairy

- ✗ Low-fat or fat-free dairy products

Opt for full-fat dairy options instead of low-fat or fat-free versions.

8. Sugary Beverages

- ✗ Soda
- ✗ Sweetened teas
- ✗ Fruit juices

9. Trans Fats

- ✗ Foods containing trans fats, often found in fried and processed foods

10. Alcohol

Limit alcohol consumption, as it can hinder ketosis and include unnecessary carbs.

11. Artificial Sweeteners

- ✗ Aspartame
- ✗ Saccharin
- ✗ Sucralose

12. Processed Meats

- ✗ Sausages with added sugar or fillers
- ✗ Processed deli meats with added sugars

13. High-Carb Sauces and Condiments

- ✗ Ketchup (often high in sugar)
- ✗ Salad dressings with added sugars
- ✗ Barbecue sauce (often high in sugar)

14. High-Sugar Snack Bars:

- ✗ Snack bars labeled as "healthy" but containing high sugar content

15. Baked Goods

- ✗ Cakes
- ✗ Cookies
- ✗ Pastries
- ✗ Breads (non-keto varieties)

16. High-Carb Nuts and Seeds

- ✗ Cashews (higher in carbs compared to other nuts)
- ✗ Peanuts (legumes, not nuts)

Chapter 5: Exercise and Fitness for Seniors on a Ketogenic Diet

5.1 Physical Activity for Healthy Aging

Incorporating physical activity into your lifestyle is crucial for healthy aging, particularly for seniors following a ketogenic diet. Regular exercise not only complements the principles of the ketogenic lifestyle but also amplifies its benefits, contributing significantly to your overall well-being. As we age, maintaining muscle mass and strength becomes increasingly vital for everyday activities and independence. Incorporating resistance training into your fitness routine, such as weightlifting or resistance band exercises, can effectively preserve muscle mass and function, supporting your mobility and autonomy. Cardiovascular health is paramount for seniors, and engaging in activities like brisk walking, swimming, or cycling can significantly improve heart health and overall fitness. These exercises enhance cardiovascular function, reduce the risk of heart disease, and bolster endurance, even with low-impact options that are gentle on aging joints. Flexibility and mobility often decline with age, but incorporating stretching exercises into your routine can counteract stiffness and reduce the risk of injury. Gentle yoga or dedicated stretching sessions can improve flexibility, allowing for greater range of motion and ease of movement. Maintaining balance and coordination is crucial for preventing falls and maintaining stability as you age. Balance exercises like standing on one leg or practicing Tai Chi can improve equilibrium and reduce the risk of accidents, promoting confidence and independence. Exercising on a ketogenic diet encourages your body to efficiently use ketones for energy, leading to improved endurance during workouts. However, it's essential to stay hydrated and maintain electrolyte balance to support your body's performance during exercise. Consistency is key when it comes to reaping the benefits of physical activity. Establishing a regular exercise routine that includes a variety of exercises, such as strength training, cardiovascular activities, flexibility work, and balance exercises, ensures that you maintain overall health and vitality as a senior on the keto diet.

Benefits of Physical Activity for Seniors on the Keto Diet

Regular physical activity holds numerous advantages for seniors, especially those following a ketogenic lifestyle. These benefits span beyond mere physical health and encompass various aspects of overall well-being. Let's delve into the positive impacts of maintaining an active lifestyle:

- ✓ **Enhanced Physical Health:** Engaging in regular exercise contributes to improved cardiovascular health, lowering the risk of chronic conditions such as heart disease and diabetes. It also boosts overall physical fitness, aiding in weight management and supporting joint health essential for mobility.

- ✓ **Increased Energy Levels:** Contrary to common belief, physical activity doesn't deplete energy but rather enhances it. By facilitating the circulation of oxygen and nutrients throughout the body, exercise leaves seniors feeling more energized and mentally alert.

✓ **Improved Mental Well-Being:** Exercise profoundly affects mental health by reducing symptoms of anxiety and depression, elevating mood, and fostering feelings of happiness and relaxation. It also bolsters cognitive function and memory, promoting mental sharpness in seniors.

✓ **Enhanced Quality of Life:** An active lifestyle contributes to an overall higher quality of life, enabling seniors to tackle daily activities with greater ease, maintain independence, and pursue hobbies and interests. Remaining physically active fosters fulfillment and enjoyment in the senior years.

✓ **Social Interaction:** Participating in group activities or classes provides opportunities for social interaction and community engagement. Connecting with others who share similar interests helps combat feelings of isolation and loneliness commonly experienced by seniors.

✓ **Better Sleep:** Participating in group activities or classes provides opportunities for social interaction and community engagement. Connecting with others who share similar interests helps combat feelings of isolation and loneliness commonly experienced by seniors.

5.2 Precautions for Physical Activity in Seniors on the Keto Diet

While physical activity offers numerous benefits, taking precautions is essential, especially for seniors following a ketogenic lifestyle. Here are some important considerations to ensure safe and enjoyable exercise experiences:

✓ **Consult with a Healthcare Provider:** Before starting a new exercise regimen, consult with your healthcare provider to assess your health status and identify any limitations or concerns. Their guidance can help tailor an exercise plan suited to your needs.

✓ **Choose Appropriate Activities:** Select activities suitable for your fitness level and needs, such as low-impact exercises like walking, swimming, or gentle yoga, which provide benefits while being gentle on the joints.

✓ **Warm-Up and Cool Down:** Always include warm-up and cool-down periods to prepare your body for activity and reduce the risk of injury. Incorporating stretching exercises can improve flexibility and prevent muscle strain..

✓ **Stay Hydrated:** Ensure adequate hydration by drinking water before, during, and after workouts, particularly in warm weather, to prevent dehydration.

✓ **Listen to Your Body:** Pay attention to your body's signals during exercise, stopping immediately if you experience pain, dizziness, or unusual symptoms. Exercise at a pace comfortable for you to avoid overexertion.

✓ **Balance and Coordination:** Include exercises focusing on balance and coordination to prevent falls and maintain stability, enhancing overall safety during physical activity.

✓ **Rest and Recovery:** Allow sufficient time for rest and recovery between workouts to prevent overexertion and optimize muscle recovery, particularly as you age.

- ✓ **Nutritional Adequacy:** Ensure your ketogenic diet provides sufficient nutrients to support physical activity, including protein, vitamins, and minerals crucial for muscle health and overall well-being.

- ✓ **Gradual Progression:** Start your exercise routine gradually and progress slowly to avoid overexertion, gradually increasing intensity and duration as your fitness improves.

- ✓ **Proper Footwear:** Choose supportive and comfortable footwear appropriate for your chosen activities to minimize discomfort and reduce the risk of injuries.

- ✓ **Joint Care**: Pay attention to joint health by engaging in low-impact exercises and seeking guidance from healthcare providers if experiencing joint pain.

- ✓ **Regular Monitoring:** Keep track of your exercise activities and progress over time to stay motivated and identify changes in fitness level, sharing this information with your healthcare provider.

- ✓ **Safety Measures:** Exercise in a safe environment using proper equipment, maintaining good posture, and being aware of surroundings to prevent accidents.

- ✓ **Consultation:** Maintain open communication with your healthcare provider, discussing any concerns or modifications needed in your exercise routine.

- ✓ **Social Support:** Engage in physical activities with others whenever possible to boost motivation, social interaction, and enjoyment, enhancing the sustainability of your exercise routine.

- ✓ **Adaptation:** Be adaptable and willing to modify your exercise routine to accommodate any physical changes associated with aging while still remaining active and engaged.

Remember, prioritizing safety and individualization is crucial when combining a ketogenic diet with physical activity in your senior years. Always prioritize your health and well-being, seeking guidance from healthcare professionals or fitness experts as needed to create a tailored and safe exercise plan.

5.3 21-Day Exercise Plan For Women (Compatible with Keto Lifestyle)

Here's a 21-day exercise plan designed specifically for women seniors following a ketogenic lifestyle. These exercises are beginner-friendly and can be done at your own pace.

Week 1: Getting Started

- ➤ **Day 1: 10-min gentle walk.** Begin with a slow-paced walk around your neighborhood or in a park. Maintain a comfortable pace.

- ➤ **Day 2: 10-min stretching routine.** Perform gentle stretching exercises for major muscle groups, holding each stretch for around 20 secs.

- ➤ **Day 3: 15-min balance exercises.** Stand on one leg for 10 secs, then switch to the other leg. Repeat this several times to improve balance.

- ➤ **Day 4: 10-min gentle walk.** Similar to Day 1, take a leisurely walk at your own pace.

- ➢ **Day 5: 10-min stretching routine.** Repeat the stretching routine from Day 2.
- ➢ **Day 6: 15-min bodyweight exercises.** Try simple bodyweight exercises like squats (slowly lower and raise your body) and wall push-ups (standing push-ups against a wall).
- ➢ **Day 7: Rest day**

Week 2: Building Stamina

- ➢ **Day 8: 15-min gentle walk.** Smildly increase your walking time from Day 4.
- ➢ **Day 9: 10-min stretching routine.** Repeat the stretching routine from Day 2.
- ➢ **Day 10: 20-min balance exercises and light resistance band exercises.** Use a resistance band for exercises like seated leg lifts and seated rows. Balance exercises include standing on one leg with your eyes closed.
- ➢ **Day 11: 15-min gentle walk.** Similar to Day 8, continue building walking endurance.
- ➢ **Day 12: 10-min stretching routine.** Repeat the stretching routine from Day 2.
- ➢ **Day 13: 20-min bodyweight exercises and light resistance band exercises.** Continue bodyweight exercises and resistance band exercises, including seated leg lifts, wall push-ups, and seated rows.
- ➢ **Day 14: Rest day**

Week 3: Progression

- ➢ **Day 15: 20-min gentle walk.** Smildly increase your walking time from Day 11.
- ➢ **Day 16: 15-min stretching routine.** Repeat the stretching routine from Day 2.
- ➢ **Day 17: 25-min balance exercises, light resistance band exercises, and gentle yoga.** Incorporate more balance exercises, resistance band exercises, and gentle yoga poses like the cat-cow stretch.
- ➢ **Day 18: 20-min gentle walk.** Similar to Day 15, continue building walking endurance.
- ➢ **Day 19: 15-min stretching routine.** Repeat the stretching routine from Day 2.
- ➢ **Day 20: 25-min bodyweight exercises, light resistance band exercises, and gentle yoga.** Continue with bodyweight exercises, resistance band exercises, and gentle yoga, including poses like the child's pose.
- ➢ **Day 21: Rest day**

Summary Of Practical Tips:

- ✓ Start each session with a warm-up and end with a cool-down.
- ✓ Listen to your body and modify exercises as needed.
- ✓ Stay hydrated throughout your workouts.
- ✓ Incorporate relaxation techniques like deep breathing after your sessions.
- ✓ Track your progress and celebrate small achievements.

Remember, the key is consistency and gradual progression. Adjust the plan to your comfort level, and enjoy the journey to improved fitness and well-being.

5.4 21-Day Exercise Plan For Men (Compatible with Keto Lifestyle)

Here's a 21-day exercise plan tailored specifically for men seniors following a ketogenic lifestyle. These exercises are designed to be beginner-friendly and adaptable to individual fitness levels.

Week 1: Getting Started

- ➤ **Day 1: 10-minute brisk walk.** Start with a brisk walk to get your heart rate up and increase circulation.

- ➤ **Day 2: 10-minute dynamic stretching routine.** Perform dynamic stretches to warm up your muscles and joints, such as leg swings, arm circles, and torso twists.

- ➤ **Day 3: 5-minute strength training.** Focus on bodyweight exercises like squats, lunges, push-ups, and plank holds to build muscle and improve functional strength.

- ➤ **Day 4: 10-minute moderate-intensity cardio.** Choose an activity like cycling, swimming, or using an elliptical machine to get your heart pumping..

- ➤ **Day 5: 10-minute yoga or mobility routine.** Incorporate gentle yoga poses or mobility exercises to improve flexibility and joint mobility.

- ➤ **Day 6: 15-minute resistance band workout.** Use resistance bands for exercises like bicep curls, shoulder presses, rows, and tricep extensions to target different muscle groups.

- ➤ **Day 7: Rest day**

Week 2: Building Stamina

- ➤ **Day 8: 15-minute brisk walk.** Increase the intensity of your walk to challenge your cardiovascular system.

- ➤ **Day 9: 10-minute dynamic stretching routine.**

- ➤ **Day 10: 20-minute strength training.** Add more challenging variations of bodyweight exercises or incorporate light dumbbells for added resistance.

- ➤ **Day 11: 15-minute moderate-intensity cardio.**

- ➤ **Day 12: 10-minute yoga or mobility routine.**

- ➤ **Day 13: 20-minute resistance band workout.** Increase the resistance or try more advanced band exercises.

- ➤ **Day 14: Rest day**

Week 3: Progression

- ➤ **Day 15: 20-minute brisk walk.**

- ➤ **Day 16: 15-minute dynamic stretching routine.**

- ➤ **Day 17: 25-minute strength training.** Focus on compound exercises that target multiple muscle groups simultaneously.

- ➤ **Day 18: 20-minute moderate-intensity cardio.**

- ➤ **Day 19: 15-minute yoga or mobility routine..**

- ➤ **Day 20: 25-minute resistance band workout.** Challenge yourself with heavier resistance bands or more repetitions.

- ➤ **Day 21: Rest day**

Remember to adjust the intensity and duration of exercises based on your fitness level and any pre-existing health conditions. Stay hydrated, listen to your body, and consult with a healthcare provider before starting any new exercise program.

5.5 21-Day Exercise Plan For Seniors (Compatible with Keto Lifestyle)

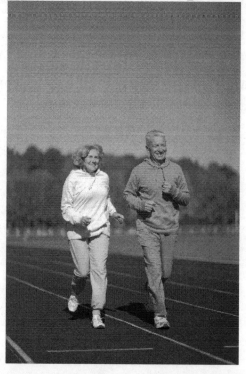

This 21-day exercise plan is designed for seniors following a ketogenic lifestyle, regardless of gender. Whether you're looking to exercise with your partner or simply seeking a balanced fitness routine, this plan offers a variety of exercises suitable for both men and women. Each session is carefully crafted to promote mobility, strength, balance, and overall well-being.

Week 1: Getting Started

- ➤ **Day 1: 10-min gentle walk:** Begin with a leisurely stroll to ease into your fitness routine.

- ➤ **Day 2: 10-min stretching routine:** Perform gentle stretches to improve flexibility and prevent injury.

- ➢ **Day 3: 15-min balance exercises:** Practice standing on one leg to enhance balance and stability.
- ➢ **Day 4: 10-min gentle walk:** Continue with another short walk to build endurance.
- ➢ **Day 5: 10-min stretching routine:** Repeat stretching exercises to maintain flexibility.
- ➢ **Day 6: 15-min bodyweight exercises:** Incorporate squats and wall push-ups to build strength.
- ➢ **Day 7: Rest day:** Allow your body to recover and prepare for the week ahead.

Week 2: Building Stamina

- ➢ **Day 8: 15-min gentle walk**: Increase walking time slightly to challenge yourself.
- ➢ **Day 9: 10-min stretching routine:** Stretch major muscle groups to prevent stiffness.
- ➢ **Day 10: 20-min light resistance band exercises:** Use resistance bands for seated leg lifts and rows to tone muscles.
- ➢ **Day 11: 15-min gentle walk:** Maintain consistency with another walk to boost cardiovascular health.
- ➢ **Day 12: 10-min stretching routine:** Continue stretching to improve flexibility and range of motion.
- ➢ **Day 13: 20-min bodyweight exercises:** Perform lunges and bicep curls with light weights to build muscle.
- ➢ **Day 14: Rest day:** Take a day off to rest and recharge.

Week 3: Progression

- ➢ **Day 15: 20-min gentle walk:** Extend your walking time to challenge yourself further.
- ➢ **Day 16: 15-min stretching routine:** Stretching helps prevent injury and promotes relaxation.
- ➢ **Day 17: 25-min balance exercises and gentle yoga:** Practice balance exercises and gentle yoga poses like the cat-cow stretch for flexibility.
- ➢ **Day 18: 20-min gentle walk:** Keep up the momentum with another walk to stay active.
- ➢ **Day 19: 15-min stretching routine:** Focus on deep stretches to release tension in muscles.
- ➢ **Day 20: 25-min bodyweight exercises and light resistance band exercises:** Incorporate chest presses and tricep extensions for upper body strength.
- ➢ **Day 21: Rest day:** Reflect on your progress and give your body the rest it deserves.

Chapter 6: Keto Recipes For Breakfast

1. Creamy Avocado and Smoked Salmon Toast

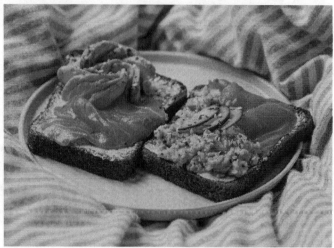

(Setup Time: 5 mins | Cooked in: 2 mins | How Many People: 2)

This delightful breakfast recipe combines the richness of avocado with the savory goodness of smoked salmon, making it a perfect choice for seniors following a ketogenic diet. Avocado is a nutrient-dense fruit rich in heart-healthy monounsaturated fats, fiber, vitamins, and minerals. Its creamy texture adds a satisfying element to this dish while providing essential nutrients. Smoked salmon is an excellent source of protein and omega-3 fatty acids, which are beneficial for heart health and inflammation reduction. The addition of cream cheese not only enhances the creaminess but also contributes to the overall flavor profile of the toast. This recipe is quick and easy to prepare, requiring minimal setup time. It offers a well-balanced combination of macronutrients, with moderate protein and low carbohydrates, making it suitable for seniors looking to maintain stable blood sugar levels and promote ketosis.

Recipe Components:

- 1 ripe avocado
- 2 slices of your choice of bread (e.g., whole grain, sourdough)
- 100g (3.5 oz) smoked salmon
- 2 tbsps cream cheese
- 1 lemon
- Salt and pepper as required
- Fresh dill for garnish (optional)

Preparation Steps: Toast the bread slices till they are golden brown to your liking. While the bread is toasting, cut the ripe avocado in half, take out the pit, and scoop out the flesh into a container. Squeeze the juice of half a lemon into the container with the avocado. Mash the avocado and lemon juice together till you achieve a creamy consistency. Season the avocado mixture with a tweak of salt and pepper as required. Once the toast is ready, spread a tbsp of cream cheese on each slice. Top the cream cheese with the creamy avocado mixture. Lay slices of smoked salmon on top of the avocado. Garnish with fresh dill if wanted.

Nutritional Info: Calories: 388 kcal, Protein: 4.9g, Carb: 12.7g, Fat: 33.4g.

2. Blueberry Chia Pudding

(Setup Time: 5 mins plus refrigeration time | How Many People: 2)

This Blueberry Chia Pudding offers a delightful blend of flavors and textures, making it an ideal breakfast option for seniors following a ketogenic diet. Chia seeds are the star ingredient, providing a rich source of omega-3 fatty acids, fiber, and antioxidants. When combined with unsweetened almond milk, they create a creamy pudding-like consistency that is both satisfying and nutritious. Fresh blueberries not only add a burst of sweetness but also contribute vitamins, minerals, and additional antioxidants to the dish. Blueberries are known for their anti-inflammatory properties and may help support cognitive function, making them particularly beneficial for seniors. The addition of vanilla extract and maple syrup or honey enhances the flavor profile of the pudding without compromising its keto-friendly nature. Seniors can adjust the sweetness to their preference while still enjoying a delicious and wholesome breakfast option. This recipe is quick and easy to prepare, requiring minimal setup time. By refrigerating the pudding for a few hours or overnight, seniors can ensure that the chia seeds absorb the liquid and create the desired consistency.

Recipe Components:

- 1/4 teacup chia seeds
- 1 teacup unsweetened almond milk (or any milk of your choice)
- 1/2 tsp vanilla extract
- 1 tbsp maple syrup or honey (adjust as required)
- 1/2 teacup fresh blueberries
- Fresh mint leaves for garnish (optional)

Preparation Steps: Inside a blending container, blend the chia seeds, almond milk, vanilla extract, and maple syrup or honey. Stir the mixture thoroughly, making sure the chia seeds are well distributed. Cover the container and put in the fridge it for almost 2 hrs or overnight to allow the chia seeds to absorb the liquid and create a pudding-like consistency. Before presenting, give the pudding a good stir to ensure it's smooth. Split the pudding into two presenting glasses. Top each presenting with fresh blueberries and garnish with mint leaves if wanted.

Nutritional Info: Calories: 210 kcal, Protein: 5g, Carb: 22g, Fat: 11g, Fiber: 11g, Sugar: 7g.

3. Spinach and Mushroom Breakfast Casserole

(Setup Time: 15 mins | Cooked in: 45 mins | How Many People: 6-8)

This Spinach and Mushroom Breakfast Casserole is a hearty and nutritious dish that's perfect for seniors following a ketogenic diet. Packed with protein-rich eggs and savory vegetables like spinach, mushrooms, and onions, this casserole provides a satisfying and flavorful breakfast option. Eggs are a fantastic source of high-quality protein, essential vitamins, and minerals, making them an excellent choice for seniors looking to maintain muscle mass and support overall health. The addition of spinach adds a dose of vitamins A and K, as well as antioxidants that may help reduce inflammation and support immune function. Meanwhile, mushrooms contribute additional vitamins and minerals, including vitamin D, which is essential for bone health.

Shredded cheddar cheese not only adds creaminess and flavor but also provides calcium and protein. Calcium is vital for maintaining bone health, especially for seniors who may be at risk of osteoporosis. With minimal preparation time and simple ingredients, this casserole is easy to make and can be prepared ahead of time for busy mornings. Seniors can enjoy a satisfying breakfast that keeps them full and energized throughout the day while staying within their ketogenic macros. Each serving of this Spinach and Mushroom Breakfast Casserole is packed with nutrients, offering a balanced combination of protein, healthy fats, and fiber. It's a delicious and wholesome option for seniors looking to kickstart their day on a nutritious note while adhering to their ketogenic lifestyle.

Recipe Components:

- 8 big eggs
- 1 teacup milk
- 1 (10 oz) package frozen severed spinach, thawed and drained
- 1 teacup carved mushrooms
- 1/2 teacup cubed onion
- 1 1/2 teacups shredded cheddar cheese
- Salt and pepper as required

Preparation Steps: Warm up your oven to 350 deg.F (175 deg.C) and grease a 9x13-inch baking dish. Inside a big blending container, whisk collectively the eggs and milk. Include the thawed and drained spinach, carved mushrooms, cubed onion, and 1 teacup of shredded cheddar cheese to the egg mixture. Season with salt and pepper as required, then mix everything thoroughly. Pour the mixture into the prepared baking dish. Spray the rest of the 1/2 teacup of shredded cheddar cheese on top. Bake in the warmed up oven for around 45 mins or till the casserole is set and the top is golden brown. Allow it to cool for a couple of mins before presenting. Cut into squares and serve your Spinach and Mushroom Breakfast Casserole.

Nutritional Info: Serving size: 1 square (assuming 8 presentings) - Calories: 175 kcal, Protein: 12g, Carb: 6g, Fat: 11g.

4. Cauliflower Hash Browns

(Setup Time: 15 mins | Cooked in: 20 mins | How Many People: 4)

These Cauliflower Hash Browns offer a delicious and keto-friendly twist on a classic breakfast favorite, perfect for seniors looking to enjoy a flavorful and satisfying meal. Made with nutritious cauliflower as the base, these hash browns are low in carbohydrates and packed with essential vitamins and minerals. Cauliflower is rich in antioxidants, fiber, and vitamins C and K, making it an excellent choice for supporting overall health and well-being in seniors. By replacing traditional potatoes with cauliflower, these hash browns are lower in carbs and calories while still delivering a crispy and satisfying texture. Plus, cauliflower is known for its versatility, allowing you to enjoy your favorite comfort foods without sacrificing flavor or nutrition. The addition of parmesan and cheddar cheese adds a deliciously cheesy flavor and provides calcium and protein, essential nutrients for bone health and muscle maintenance in seniors. Almond flour serves as a gluten-free and low-carb alternative to traditional wheat flour, adding a nutty flavor and helping to bind the ingredients together.

With just a few simple ingredients and minimal prep time, these Cauliflower Hash Browns are easy to make and can be enjoyed as part of a balanced ketogenic breakfast. Seniors can indulge in a hearty and flavorful meal without worrying about compromising their dietary goals.

Recipe Components:

- 1 small cauliflower head, cut into florets
- 1/4 teacup grated parmesan cheese
- 1/4 teacup shredded cheddar cheese
- 1/4 teacup almond flour
- 1 big egg
- 1/2 tsp garlic powder
- 1/2 tsp onion powder
- Salt and pepper as required
- Cooking spray or oil for frying

Preparation Steps: Begin by preheating your oven to 425 deg.F (220 deg.C) and placing a baking sheet with parchment paper. Inside a food processor, pulse the cauliflower florets till they resemble rice. Transfer the cauliflower rice to a microwave-safe container and microwave for 5 mins. Allow the microwaved cauliflower to cool and then use a clean kitchen towel to squeeze out excess moisture. Inside a blending container, blend the cauliflower, parmesan cheese, cheddar cheese, almond flour, egg, garlic powder, onion powder, salt, and pepper. Mix till all components are thoroughly mixed. Split the mixture into 4 equal portions and shape them into oval-shaped patties. Heat a griddle at med-high temp. and mildly grease with cooking spray or oil. Cook the cauliflower hash browns for around 4-5 mins on all sides, or till they are golden brown and crispy. Transfer them to the prepared baking sheet and finish baking in the oven for an extra 10 mins to ensure they are fully cooked. Serve your Cauliflower Hash Browns hot and enjoy.

Nutritional Info: Calories: 127 kcal, Protein: 7g, Carb: 7g, Fat: 9g.

5. Coconut Almond Keto Pancakes

(Setup Time: 10 mins | Cooked in: 10 mins | How Many People: 2)

These pancakes are not only delicious but also keto-friendly, offering a satisfying alternative to traditional high-carb breakfast options. Made with wholesome ingredients like almond flour and coconut flour, these pancakes are low in carbs and high in healthy fats, making them an ideal choice for seniors looking to maintain ketosis. Almond flour provides a rich source of protein, fiber, and essential nutrients, including vitamin E and magnesium, which are beneficial for heart health and overall well-being in seniors. Coconut flour adds a subtle sweetness and a hint of tropical flavor to these pancakes while contributing healthy fats and dietary fiber. With just a few simple ingredients and minimal prep time, these Coconut Almond Keto Pancakes are easy to whip up, allowing seniors to enjoy a delicious breakfast without spending hours in the kitchen. Each serving of these pancakes is packed with protein and healthy fats, providing sustained energy and keeping you feeling full and satisfied throughout the morning. Plus, they're customizable with your favorite keto-friendly toppings, such as sugar-free syrup, fresh berries, or whipped cream, allowing you to indulge in a variety of flavors while staying true to your dietary goals.

Recipe Components:

- 1/2 teacup almond flour
- 2 tbsps coconut flour
- 1/2 tsp baking powder
- 2 big eggs
- 1/4 teacup unsweetened almond milk
- 2 tbsps coconut oil, dissolved
- 1/2 tsp vanilla extract
- 1-2 tbsps erythritol or your preferred keto-friendly sweetener (adjust as required)
- Pinch of salt

Preparation Steps: Inside a blending container, blend the almond flour, coconut flour, baking powder, and a tweak of salt. Inside a distinct container, whisk the eggs, almond milk, dissolved coconut oil, vanilla extract, and sweetener. Pour the wet components into the dry components and mix till a smooth batter forms. Heat a non-stick griddle or griddle at med temp. and mildly grease it with coconut oil. Pour 1/4 teacup of the batter onto the griddle to form each pancake. Cook for 2-3 mins on all sides, or till they are golden brown and fully cooked. Repeat the process till the entire batter is utilized. Serve your Coconut Almond Keto Pancakes with your choice of keto-friendly toppings like sugar-free syrup, berries, or whipped cream.

Nutritional Info: Calories: 330 kcal, Protein: 12g, Carb: 11g, Fiber: 6g, Net Carbs: 5g, Fat: 26g.

6. Cheddar and Chive Keto Biscuits

(Setup Time: 10 mins | Cooked in: 20 mins | How Many People: 6)

These biscuits are a delicious and nutritious option for breakfast or as a side dish, offering a satisfying alternative to traditional high-carb biscuits. Made with almond flour and coconut flour, they are low in carbs and packed with healthy fats, making them suitable for seniors looking to maintain ketosis while enjoying their favorite baked goods. Almond flour provides a rich source of protein and essential nutrients, including vitamin E and magnesium, which are beneficial for heart health and overall well-being in seniors. Coconut flour adds a hint of sweetness and a light, fluffy texture to these biscuits while contributing dietary fiber to support digestive health. The addition of sharp cheddar cheese and finely chopped chives adds savory flavor and aromatic freshness to these biscuits, elevating them to a gourmet level. Each bite is bursting with cheesy goodness and herbal notes, making them a delightful treat for the taste buds. With just a few simple ingredients and minimal prep time, these Cheddar and Chive Keto Biscuits are easy to make and perfect for seniors looking to enjoy a wholesome and satisfying meal. Whether served warm from the oven or enjoyed as a convenient grab-and-go snack, these biscuits are sure to become a favorite among seniors following a ketogenic diet. Each biscuit is packed with protein, healthy fats, and dietary fiber, providing sustained energy and keeping you feeling full and satisfied throughout the day. Plus, they're versatile enough to pair with a variety of dishes or enjoy on their own as a delicious and nutritious snack.

Recipe Components:

- 1 1/2 teacups almond flour
- 1/4 teacup coconut flour
- 1 1/2 tsps baking powder
- 1/2 tsp garlic powder
- 1/4 tsp salt
- 1/4 teacup chives, finely severed
- 1 1/2 teacups shredded sharp cheddar cheese

- 1/2 teacup unsalted butter, dissolved
- 3 big eggs

Preparation Steps: Warm up your oven to 350 deg.F (175 deg.C) and line a baking sheet with parchment paper. Inside a blending container, blend the almond flour, coconut flour, baking powder, garlic powder, and salt. Stir in the finely severed chives and shredded cheddar cheese. Inside a distinct container, whisk the dissolved butter and eggs together. Pour the wet mixture into the dry components and stir till you have a dense dough. Use your hands to form 6 equal-sized biscuit rounds and place them on the prepared baking sheet. Bake in the warmed up oven for around 20 mins or till the biscuits are golden brown and firm to the touch. Allow the biscuits to cool for a couple of mins before presenting.

Nutritional Info: Calories: 415 kcal, Protein: 13g, Carb: 9g, Fiber: 4g, Net Carbs: 5g, Fat: 37g.

7. Turmeric Scrambled Eggs

(Setup Time: 5 mins | Cooked in: 5 mins | How Many People: 2)

These scrambled eggs are infused with aromatic spices like ground turmeric, cumin, and coriander, adding a burst of flavor and a vibrant golden hue to your morning meal. Turmeric, in particular, is known for its anti-inflammatory properties and potential health benefits, making it an excellent addition to a senior's diet. Combined with protein-rich eggs, this dish provides a satisfying and nourishing start to the day. Whisked together with ground spices, salt, and pepper, these scrambled eggs are cooked to perfection in butter or ghee, resulting in a creamy and decadent texture that melts in your mouth. The addition of fresh cilantro adds a pop of color and a refreshing herbal note, enhancing the overall flavor profile of the dish. Not only are these Turmeric Scrambled Eggs delicious, but they're also packed with essential nutrients, including protein and healthy fats, to keep you feeling full and energized throughout the morning.

Recipe Components:

- 4 big eggs
- 1/2 tsp ground turmeric
- 1/4 tsp ground cumin
- 1/4 tsp ground coriander
- Salt and pepper as required
- 2 tbsps butter or ghee
- Fresh cilantro for garnish (optional)

Preparation Steps: Inside a container, whisk the eggs till well beaten. Include the ground turmeric, ground cumin, ground coriander, salt, and pepper to the beaten eggs. Whisk everything together till the spices are well incorporated. Heat the butter or ghee in a non-stick griddle at med temp. Pour the spiced egg mixture into the griddle. Stir continuously with a spatula for around 3-4 mins till the eggs are fully cooked and mildly creamy. Once cooked to your anticipated uniformity, take out from heat. Garnish with fresh cilantro if wanted.

Nutritional Info: Calories: 236 kcal, Protein: 12g, Carb: 1g, Fat: 20g.

8. Keto Strawberry Smoothie Bowl

(Setup Time: 5 mins | How Many People: 1)

Crafted with carefully selected ingredients, this smoothie bowl offers a burst of flavor and a wealth of health benefits to kickstart your day. Frozen strawberries serve as the star ingredient, providing a sweet and tangy taste while contributing essential vitamins and antioxidants to support overall health. Blended with unsweetened almond milk and Greek yogurt, this smoothie bowl achieves a creamy and satisfying texture without compromising on keto-friendly principles. Chia seeds add a nutritious boost of fiber, omega-3 fatty acids, and protein, promoting digestive health and satiety. Enhanced with a touch of vanilla extract and erythritol, a keto-friendly sweetener, this smoothie bowl offers just the right amount of sweetness without spiking blood sugar levels, making it an ideal choice for seniors looking to maintain stable energy levels throughout the day. Topped with sliced strawberries, chia seeds, unsweetened coconut flakes, and carved almonds, this smoothie bowl is as visually appealing as it is delicious, adding a delightful crunch and texture to each bite. With only five minutes of setup time, this Keto Strawberry Smoothie Bowl is a quick and convenient breakfast option that's perfect for busy mornings. Whether enjoyed as a refreshing start to your day or as a satisfying midday snack, this smoothie bowl is sure to satisfy your cravings while keeping you on track with your keto goals.

Recipe Components:

- 1 teacup frozen strawberries
- 1/2 teacup unsweetened almond milk
- 1/4 teacup Greek yogurt
- 1 tbsp chia seeds
- 1/2 tsp vanilla extract
- 1/2 tsp erythritol (or your preferred keto-friendly sweetener)
- Toppings: Sliced strawberries, chia seeds, unsweetened coconut flakes, and carved almonds (optional)

Preparation Steps: Inside a blender, blend the frozen strawberries, unsweetened almond milk, Greek yogurt, chia seeds, vanilla extract, and erythritol. Blend till the mixture is smooth and creamy. Pour the smoothie into a container. Top with carved strawberries, chia seeds, unsweetened coconut flakes, and carved almonds if wanted.

Nutritional Info: Cal: 240 kcal, Protein: 8g, Carb: 20g (Net Carbs: 8g), Fiber: 12g, Fat: 14g

9. Bacon-Wrapped Asparagus

(Setup Time: 10 mins | Cooked in: 20 mins | How Many People: 4)

With just a handful of ingredients and minimal preparation time, this recipe offers a delightful combination of flavors and textures that are sure to tantalize your taste buds. Fresh asparagus spears serve as the nutritious centerpiece, providing a rich source of vitamins, minerals, and antioxidants to support overall health and well-being. Each spear is carefully enveloped in savory bacon slices, adding a touch of smokiness and indulgence to every bite. The crispy texture of the bacon perfectly complements the tender-crisp asparagus, creating a harmonious balance of flavors that is both satisfying and delicious.

Enhanced with a drizzle of olive oil and a sprinkle of salt and pepper, these Bacon-Wrapped Asparagus bundles are roasted to perfection in the oven, allowing the flavors to meld together and the bacon to crisp up beautifully. Ideal for breakfast, brunch, or as a flavorful side dish, these bacon-wrapped bundles are as visually appealing as they are delicious, making them a standout addition to any meal. Plus, with each serving containing just 4 grams of carbs, you can enjoy this dish guilt-free while staying true to your keto goals.

Recipe Components:

- 1 bunch of asparagus spears (about 16 spears)
- 8 slices of bacon
- 1 tbsp olive oil
- Salt and pepper as required

Preparation Steps: Warm up your oven to 400 deg.F (200 deg.C). Wash and trim the woody ends of the asparagus spears. Split the asparagus into bundles of 4 spears each. Wrap each bundle with 2 slices of bacon, securing the ends with toothpicks. Put the bacon-wrapped asparagus bundles on a baking sheet, spray with olive oil, and season with salt and pepper. Roast in the warmed up oven for around 20 mins or till the bacon is crispy, and the asparagus is soft. Take out the toothpicks before presenting.

Nutritional Info: Calories: 160 kcal, Protein: 5g, Carb: 4g, Fiber: 2g, Fat: 14g

10. Almond Flour Waffles

(Setup Time: 10 mins | Cooked in: 15 mins | How Many People: 4)

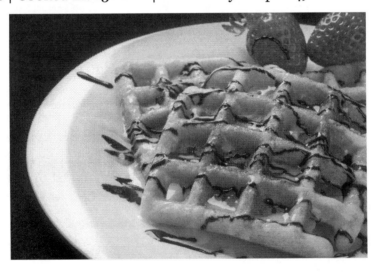

These waffles offer a perfect balance of flavor and nutrition, starting with almond flour as the primary ingredient. Almond flour not only adds a rich, nutty taste but also provides a host of health benefits, including a good source of healthy fats, protein, and fiber. Sweetened with erythritol, a low-carb sweetener, these waffles satisfy your sweet cravings without spiking blood sugar levels, making them an ideal choice for those adhering to a keto diet. With the addition of eggs, almond milk, and melted butter (or coconut oil), the batter achieves a light and fluffy texture that crisps up beautifully when cooked in a waffle iron. Each bite is a delightful combination of soft, pillowy goodness and crispy edges, creating a satisfying breakfast experience.

Versatile and customizable, these Almond Flour Waffles can be enjoyed with a variety of keto-friendly toppings, such as sugar-free syrup, fresh berries, or a dollop of whipped cream.

Recipe Components:

- 1 1/2 teacups almond flour
- 2 tbsps erythritol (or your preferred low-carb sweetener)
- 1/2 tsp baking powder
- 1/4 tsp salt
- 3 big eggs
- 1/2 teacup unsweetened almond milk
- 1/4 teacup dissolved butter or coconut oil
- 1 tsp vanilla extract

Preparation Steps: Warm up your waffle iron as per to the manufacturers guidelines. Inside a big container, whisk collectively the almond flour, erythritol, baking powder, and salt. Inside a distinct container, beat the eggs and then include the almond milk, dissolved butter (or coconut oil), and vanilla extract. Pour the wet components into the dry components and stir till thoroughly mixed. Grease the waffle iron with a little oil or cooking spray. Pour the waffle batter onto the warmed up waffle iron and cook till the waffles are golden brown and crisp. Serve the waffles with your favorite keto-friendly toppings, like sugar-free syrup or fresh berries.

Nutritional Info: Calories: 347 kcal, Protein: 11g, Carb: 8g, Fiber: 4g, Fat: 31g

11. Tomato and Basil Mini Quiches

(Setup Time: 10 mins | Cooked in: 20 mins | How Many People: 6)

With just 2 grams of carbs per serving, they offer a satisfying breakfast option that won't derail your keto goals. Each quiche is packed with protein-rich eggs and creamy heavy cream, providing essential nutrients to support overall health and satiety. Grated cheddar cheese adds a rich and savory element, while fresh basil leaves impart a fragrant aroma and subtle herbal flavor. Topped with halved cherry tomatoes, these mini quiches are as visually appealing as they are delicious. The tomatoes add a burst of vibrant color and juicy sweetness, complementing the savory flavors of the quiches. Simple to prepare, these mini quiches can be made ahead of time and stored in the refrigerator for a convenient grab-and-go breakfast option.

Recipe Components:

- 6 big eggs
- 1/2 teacup heavy cream
- 1/2 teacup grated cheddar cheese
- 1/4 teacup fresh basil leaves, severed
- 1 teacup cherry tomatoes, halved
- Salt and pepper as required

Preparation Steps: Warm up your oven to 350 deg.F (175 deg.C) and grease a muffin tin or use silicone muffin teacups. Inside a container, whisk collectively the eggs and heavy cream till thoroughly mixed. Stir in the grated cheddar cheese and severed basil leaves. Season the mixture with salt and pepper as required. Pour the egg mixture evenly into the muffin teacups, filling each about halfway. Place one halved cherry tomato on top of each quiche. Bake in the warmed up oven for around 20 mins or till the quiches are set and mildly golden on top.

Take out from the oven and let them cool for a couple of mins before presenting.

Nutritional Info: Calories: 228 kcal, Protein: 11g, Carb: 2g, Fiber: 0g, Fat: 19g

12. Mediterranean Keto Omelette
(Setup Time: 5 mins | Cooked in: 10 mins | How Many People: 2)

Loaded with nutrient-dense ingredients like spinach, tomatoes, feta cheese, and Kalamata olives, this omelette is as nourishing as it is delicious. Spinach provides a dose of vitamins and minerals, while tomatoes add a juicy sweetness and vibrant color. Tangy feta cheese and briny Kalamata olives impart a distinctive Mediterranean flair, while dried oregano adds a hint of herbal aroma. Simple to prepare and bursting with flavor, this Mediterranean Keto Omelette is the perfect way to start your day on a nutritious note. With just 5 grams of carbs per serving, it's an ideal choice for seniors looking to maintain ketosis while enjoying a flavorful and satisfying breakfast.

Recipe Components:

- 4 big eggs
- 2 tbsps heavy cream
- 1/2 teacup severed spinach
- 1/4 teacup cubed tomatoes
- 1/4 teacup crumbled feta cheese
- 2 tbsps severed Kalamata olives
- 1/4 tsp dried oregano
- Salt and pepper as required

Preparation Steps: Inside a container, whisk collectively the eggs and heavy cream till thoroughly mixed. Stir in the severed spinach, cubed tomatoes, crumbled feta cheese, and severed Kalamata olives. Season the mixture with dried oregano, salt, and pepper as required. Heat a non-stick griddle at med temp. and include a bit of cooking oil or butter. Pour half of the egg mixture into the griddle and let it cook for a couple of mins till the edges set. Gently lift the edges and tilt the griddle to let the uncooked eggs flow to the edges. When the omelette is mostly set, fold it in half and cook for an extra min till fully set. Repeat the process for the second omelette. Serve hot and garnish with additional feta, olives, and fresh oregano if wanted.

Nutritional Info: Calories: 304 kcal, Protein: 16g, Carb: 5g, Fiber: 1g, Fat: 24g

13. Keto Veggie and Cheese Frittata Muffins
(Setup Time: 10 mins | Cooked in: 20 mins | How Many People: 6)

Crafted with care and packed with wholesome ingredients, these frittata muffins are a convenient and nutritious option for breakfast or a quick snack. Each muffin is brimming with protein-rich eggs and creamy heavy cream, providing essential nutrients to fuel your day. The colorful medley of bell peppers, onions, and mushrooms adds a burst of flavor and texture to these muffins, while the shredded cheddar cheese contributes a rich and indulgent taste. Seasoned with garlic powder, salt, and pepper, these frittata muffins are perfectly seasoned for a satisfying culinary experience. Simple to prepare and bursting with flavor, these keto-friendly muffins are baked to perfection in just 20 minutes, ensuring a quick and convenient meal option for busy seniors.

Recipe Components:

- 6 big eggs
- 1/4 teacup heavy cream
- 1/2 teacup cubed bell peppers (red, green, or yellow)
- 1/4 teacup cubed onions
- 1/4 teacup cubed mushrooms
- 1/4 teacup shredded cheddar cheese
- 1/4 tsp garlic powder
- Salt and pepper as required

Preparation Steps: Warm up your oven to 350 deg.F (175 deg.C) and grease a muffin tin with cooking spray. Inside a blending container, whisk collectively the eggs and heavy cream till thoroughly mixed. Stir in the cubed bell peppers, onions, mushrooms, and shredded cheddar cheese. Season the mixture with garlic powder, salt, and pepper as required. Pour the egg and vegetable mixture evenly into the muffin tin. Bake in the warmed up oven for around 20 mins or till the frittata muffins are set and mildly golden on top. Allow them to cool for a couple of mins before removing them from the muffin tin. Serve these keto frittata muffins warm or at room tcmp.

Nutritional Info: Calories: 130 kcal, Protein: 8g, Carb: 3g, Fiber: 1g, Fat: 10g

14. Cinnamon Coconut Porridge

(Setup Time: 5 mins | Cooked in: 10 mins | How Many People: 2)

Made with unsweetened shredded coconut and creamy almond milk, this porridge is rich in healthy fats and low in carbs, making it an ideal choice for those adhering to a ketogenic diet. With just 7 grams of carbs and 200 calories per serving, it is a satisfying and nutritious option for breakfast or a comforting snack. Its rich texture and warm, aromatic spices make it a delightful treat for any time of day, providing a taste of indulgence without sacrificing your keto goals.

Recipe Components:

- 1/2 teacup unsweetened shredded coconut
- 1 teacup unsweetened almond milk (or any preferred low-carb milk)
- 2 tbsps ground flaxseed
- 1/2 tsp ground cinnamon
- 1/4 tsp vanilla extract
- Sweetener (e.g., erythritol or stevia) as required

Preparation Steps: Inside a saucepan, blend the unsweetened shredded coconut and unsweetened almond milk. Put the saucepan at med temp. and bring the mixture to a gentle simmer. Stir occasionally. Once it's simmering, decrease the temp. and let it cook for around 5 mins till it densess. Stir in the ground flaxseed, ground cinnamon, vanilla extract, and sweetener as required. Cook for an extra 2-3 mins, mixing regularly till it reaches your anticipated uniformity. Take out from heat and let it cool for a min. Serve the cinnamon coconut porridge in containers, optionally topped with extra shredded coconut and a spray of cinnamon.

Nutritional Info: Calories: 200 kcal, Protein: 3g, Carb: 7g, Fiber: 4g, Fat: 17g

15. Savory Keto Crepes

(Setup Time: 10 mins | Cooked in: 15 mins | How Many People: 2)

These crepes boast a delicate texture and savory flavor profile, making them a versatile foundation for a variety of fillings. Made with a blend of almond flour, coconut flour, eggs, and unsweetened almond milk, these crepes are low in carbs and packed with protein and healthy fats, ensuring they align perfectly with your keto goals. Their versatility allows for endless customization, making them suitable for any taste preference or dietary restriction.

Recipe Components:

- 1/2 teacup almond flour
- 2 big eggs
- 1/4 teacup unsweetened almond milk (or any preferred low-carb milk)
- 1 tbsp coconut flour

- 1/4 tsp salt
- 1/4 tsp garlic powder (optional)
- 1/4 tsp dried herbs of your choice (e.g., thyme, rosemary)
- Cooking oil or butter for greasing the pan

Preparation Steps: Inside a container, whisk collectively almond flour, coconut flour, salt, garlic powder, and dried herbs. Inside an extra container, beat the eggs and then stir in the unsweetened almond milk. Blend the wet and dry components, mixing till a smooth batter forms. Heat a non-stick griddle at med temp. and mildly grease it with oil or butter. Pour around 1/4 teacup of the batter into the griddle, swirling it around to create a thin crepe. Cook for 2-3 mins till the edges start to lift, then flip and cook for an extra 1-2 mins. Take out the crepe from the pan and repeat the process with the rest of the batter. Serve your savory keto crepes with your choice of fillings, like scrambled eggs, cheese, spinach, or smoked salmon.

Nutritional Info: Calories: 210 kcal, Protein: 10g, Carb: 6g, Fiber: 3g, Fat: 16g

16. Pecan Pie Keto Oatmeal

(Setup Time: 5 mins | Cooked in: 10 mins | How Many People: 2)

This delightful oatmeal alternative is crafted with seniors' health in mind, featuring a blend of almond flour, chia seeds, and severed pecans. Sweetened with a dash of erythritol and flavored with cinnamon and vanilla extract, this keto oatmeal provides a satisfyingly sweet taste without the need for added sugars. Rich in healthy fats and fiber, this oatmeal is gentle on the digestive system and helps seniors maintain stable energy levels throughout the day.

Plus, the inclusion of chia seeds adds an extra boost of omega-3 fatty acids, promoting heart health and cognitive function. Easy to prepare and customizable to individual preferences, this Pecan Pie Keto Oatmeal offers a warm and comforting breakfast option that seniors can enjoy guilt-free. With 330 calories per serving and a balance of protein, carbs, and fats, it's the perfect way to kickstart your morning while adhering to your keto lifestyle.

Recipe Components:

- 1/2 teacup almond flour

- 2 tbsps chia seeds

- 2 tbsps severed pecans
- 1 tbsp sweetener (e.g., erythritol or stevia)
- 1/2 tsp cinnamon
- A tweak of salt
- 1 teacup unsweetened almond milk
- 1/2 tsp vanilla extract
- 1 tbsp sugar-free maple syrup (optional, for topping)

Preparation Steps: Inside a microwave-safe container, blend almond flour, chia seeds, severed pecans, sweetener, cinnamon, and a tweak of salt. Stir in unsweetened almond milk and vanilla extract. Microwave the mixture on high for 2 mins, stopping to stir every 30 secs to prevent clumping. Allow the keto oatmeal to rest for a min or two to denses. Spray sugar-free maple syrup on top, if wanted, before presenting.

Nutritional Info: Calories: 330 kcal, Protein: 9g, Carbs: 13g, Fiber: 9g, Fat: 26g

17. Coconut Berry Parfait
(Setup Time: 10 mins | How Many People: 2)

This parfait features layers of unsweetened coconut yogurt, fresh mixed berries, and a sprinkle of unsweetened shredded coconut and severed nuts. Sweetened with a touch of stevia or erythritol and flavored with vanilla extract, this parfait offers a deliciously sweet and tangy taste without added sugars. Packed with healthy fats, antioxidants, and fiber, this parfait supports seniors' overall well-being while satisfying their sweet cravings. The Greek yogurt provides probiotics for gut health, while the berries offer vitamins and minerals to support immune function. Easy to assemble and customizable to personal preferences, this Coconut Berry Parfait is a refreshing and nutritious treat for seniors to enjoy guilt-free. With 250 calories per serving and a balance of protein, carbs, and fats, it's the perfect way to indulge in a healthy dessert or snack.

Recipe Components:

- 1 teacup unsweetened coconut yogurt
- 1/2 teacup fresh mixed berries (e.g., strawberries, blueberries, raspberries)
- 2 tbsps unsweetened shredded coconut
- 2 tbsps severed nuts (e.g., almonds or walnuts)
- 1 tbsp sugar-free sweetener (e.g., stevia or erythritol)
- 1/2 tsp vanilla extract

Preparation Steps: Inside a container, blend the unsweetened coconut yogurt with the vanilla extract and sugar-free sweetener. Mix well. In presenting glasses or containers, start by layering a spoonful of the coconut yogurt mixture. Include a layer of mixed berries on top of the yogurt. Spray a portion of the unsweetened shredded coconut and severed nuts over the berries. Repeat the layers till you fill the glasses or containers. Finish with a final spray of the coconut yogurt and a couple of berries on top for decoration. Serve instantly or put in the fridge for a refreshing and healthy dessert.

Nutritional Info: Calories: 250 kcal, Protein: 5g, Carbs: 15g, Fiber: 7g, Fat: 19g

18. Keto Zucchini Bread

(Setup Time: 15 mins | Cooked in: 50-55 mins | How Many People: 12)

Loaded with healthy fats, fiber, and vitamins, this zucchini bread supports seniors' health goals while satisfying their cravings for baked goods. The zucchini adds moisture and texture while providing essential nutrients like potassium and vitamin C. With 190 calories per serving and a balance of protein, carbs, and fats, it's a guilt-free indulgence for any time of day.

Recipe Components:

- 2 teacups almond flour
- 1/4 teacup coconut flour
- 1/4 teacup unsweetened cocoa powder
- 1 1/2 tsp baking powder
- 1/2 tsp baking soda
- 1/2 tsp salt
- 1 tsp ground cinnamon
- 1/2 teacup erythritol or preferred keto sweetener
- 1/4 teacup dissolved coconut oil
- 3 big eggs
- 1 tsp vanilla extract
- 1 1/2 teacups shredded zucchini (squeezed of excess moisture)
- 1/2 teacup sugar-free chocolate chips (optional)

Preparation Steps: Warm up your oven to 350 deg.F (175 deg.C) and grease a 9x5-inch loaf pan. Inside a big blending container, blend the almond flour, coconut flour, cocoa powder, baking powder, baking soda, salt, and ground cinnamon. Inside an extra container, whisk collectively the erythritol, dissolved coconut oil, eggs, and vanilla extract. Include the wet components to the dry components and stir till thoroughly mixed. Gently fold in the shredded zucchini and sugar-free chocolate chips if using. The batter should be poured into the prepped loaf pan and the top should be smoothed down. Bake for 50-55 mins or till a toothpick immersed into the middle comes out clean. Let the zucchini bread cool in the pan for 10 mins, then transfer it to a wire stand to cool entirely. Slice and enjoy your keto zucchini bread.

Nutritional Info: Calories: 190 kcal, Protein: 5g, Carbs: 8g, Fiber: 3g, Sugar Alcohols: 4g, Net, Carbs: 1g, Fat: 16g

19. Keto Cinnamon Roll Chaffles

(Setup Time: 5 mins | Cooked in: 10 mins | How Many People: 2)

These chaffles offer a sweet and indulgent taste without the carbs. Packed with protein and healthy fats, these chaffles provide seniors with a satisfying and nutritious meal or snack option. The addition of cinnamon adds a warm and comforting flavor while enhancing the chaffles' nutritional value. Quick and easy to make, these Keto Cinnamon Roll Chaffles are perfect for seniors looking for a delicious treat that aligns with their dietary needs. With 380 calories per serving and a balance of protein, carbs, and fats, they're a guilt-free way to enjoy a classic favorite.

Recipe Components:

- 1 big egg

- 1/2 teacup shredded mozzarella cheese
- 2 tbsps almond flour
- 1/2 tsp baking powder
- 1/2 tsp vanilla extract

- 1 tbsp erythritol or preferred keto sweetener
- 1/2 tsp ground cinnamon
- Additional butter and cinnamon for topping

For the cream cheese glaze:

- 2 tbsps cream cheese, softened
- 1 tbsp heavy cream
- 1 tbsp erythritol or preferred keto sweetener

Preparation Steps: Warm up your waffle maker. Inside a container, whisk collectively the egg, shredded mozzarella, almond flour, baking powder, vanilla extract, erythritol, and ground cinnamon. Pour half of the chaffle batter onto the warmed up waffle maker and cook for around 4-5 mins, or till it's golden and crispy. Take out the chaffle from the waffle maker and let it cool on a wire stand. Repeat with the rest of the batter to make a second chaffle. Inside a distinct container, prepare the cream cheese glaze by mixing the softened cream cheese, heavy cream, and erythritol till smooth. Disperse a layer of butter and a spray of cinnamon on one of the chaffles, then spray with the cream cheese glaze. Put the second chaffle on top to create a sandwich. Serve your keto cinnamon roll chaffle while it's warm and enjoy!

Nutritional Info: Calories: 380 kcal, Protein: 15g, Carbs: 6g, Fiber: 2g, Sugar Alcohols: 3g, Net Carbs: 1g, Fat: 32g

20. Greek Yogurt and Walnut Parfait

(Setup Time: 10 mins | How Many People: 2)

Rich in protein, healthy fats, and antioxidants, this parfait supports seniors' overall health while providing a delicious and satisfying snack option. The Greek yogurt provides probiotics for gut health, while the walnuts offer omega-3 fatty acids for heart health. Quick and easy to assemble, this Greek Yogurt and Walnut Parfait is perfect for breakfast, dessert, or snack time.

Recipe Components:

- 1 teacup Greek yogurt
- 1/4 teacup severed walnuts
- 1/4 teacup fresh blueberries

- 1 tbsp honey (optional)
- 1/4 tsp vanilla extract
- A tweak of cinnamon (optional)

Preparation Steps: Inside a container, blend Greek yogurt, vanilla extract, and honey (if wanted). Mix well. In presenting glasses or containers, start by layering a spoonful of the Greek yogurt mixture at the bottom. Include a layer of severed walnuts on top of the yogurt. Next, include a layer of fresh blueberries. Repeat the layers till the glass is filled or as desired. Finish with a dollop of Greek yogurt on top. Optionally, spray a tweak of cinnamon on the parfait for extra flavor. Serve instantly or put in the fridge for a cool and refreshing treat.

Nutritional Info: Calories: 280 kcal, Protein: 12g, Carbs: 16g, Fiber: 2g, Sugar: 10g, Fat: 20g

Chapter 7: Keto Recipes For Lunch

1. Keto Chicken and Vegetable Stir-Fry

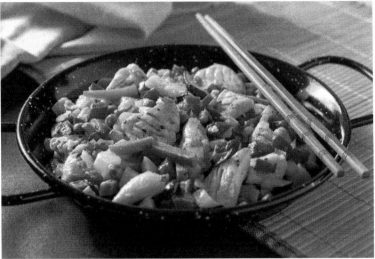

(Setup Time: 10 mins | Cooked in: 15 mins | How Many People: 4)

This flavorful dish features tender strips of chicken breast paired with an assortment of low-carb vegetables, including broccoli, bell peppers, zucchini, and snap peas. Seasoned with fresh ginger, garlic, and a dash of soy sauce, this stir-fry bursts with aromatic flavors that are gentle on the palate and satisfying to the senses. Rich in protein and essential nutrients, such as vitamins A and C, potassium, and fiber, this stir-fry provides seniors with a nourishing meal that supports overall health and well-being. Additionally, the inclusion of sesame oil adds a nutty aroma and enhances the dish's flavor profile, while natural sweeteners like erythritol provide a hint of sweetness without spiking blood sugar levels. Quick and easy to prepare, our Keto Chicken and Vegetable Stir-Fry offers a convenient lunch option that seniors can enjoy guilt-free.

Recipe Components:

- 1 lb. (450g) boneless, skinless chicken breasts, cut into fine strips
- 2 tbsps sesame oil
- 4 teacups (approx. 400g) mixed low-carb vegetables (e.g., broccoli, bell peppers, zucchini, snap peas)
- 3 pieces garlic, crushed
- 1/4 teacup (60ml) soy sauce (or tamari for gluten-free)
- 1 tbsp fresh ginger, crushed
- 2 tbsps rice vinegar
- 2 tbsps natural sweetener (e.g., erythritol or stevia)
- Salt and pepper as required
- Red pepper flakes (optional, for added heat)
- Fresh cilantro or green onions for garnish

Preparation Steps: Inside a big griddle or wok, heat 1 tbsp of sesame oil at med-high temp. Include the chicken strips and stir-fry till they're fully cooked and no longer pink in the center. Take out the chicken from the pan and put it away. Inside the same pan, include the rest of the tbsp of sesame oil. Include the crushed garlic and ginger, and sauté for around a min till fragrant. Include the mixed vegetables and stir-fry for 4-5 mins till they begin to soften.

Return the cooked chicken to the pan with the vegetables. Inside a small container, blend collectively the soy sauce, rice vinegar, sweetener, salt, and pepper. Pour this sauce over the chicken and vegetables. If you like it spicy, include red pepper flakes at this stage. Continue to stir-fry for an extra 2-3 mins, allowing the sauce to cover everything evenly. Serve hot, garnished with fresh cilantro or green onions.

Nutritional Info: Calories: 240 kcal, Protein: 25g, Carb: 7g, Fiber: 2g, Net Carbs: 5g, Fat: 12g

2. Spinach and Feta Stuffed Chicken Breast
(Setup Time: 15 mins | Cooked in: 30 mins | How Many People: 4)

High in protein and packed with essential nutrients, such as calcium, iron, and vitamins A and K, this stuffed chicken breast provides seniors with a wholesome meal that supports muscle health and overall vitality. Moreover, the inclusion of spinach adds a boost of antioxidants, while feta cheese contributes a rich and creamy texture to the filling.

Recipe Components:

- 4 boneless, skinless chicken breasts
- 1 teacup frozen spinach, thawed and drained
- 1/2 teacup feta cheese, crumbled
- 1/4 teacup cream cheese
- 1/4 teacup grated Parmesan cheese
- 2 pieces garlic, crushed
- 1 tsp dried oregano
- Salt and pepper as required
- Olive oil for cooking

Preparation Steps: Warm up your oven to 375 deg.F (190 deg.C). Inside a blending container, blend the thawed and drained spinach, crumbled feta cheese, cream cheese, grated Parmesan cheese, crushed garlic, dried oregano, salt, and pepper. Mix well to create the stuffing mixture. Slice a pocket into the side of each chicken breast. Take cautious not to sever the whole thing with your knife. Stuff each chicken breast with the spinach and cheese mixture, evenly distributing the stuffing among them. Heat some olive oil in an ovenproof griddle at med-high temp. Put the stuffed chicken breasts in the griddle and cook for 2-3 mins on all sides till they're nicely browned. Transfer the griddle to the warmed up oven and bake for around 20-25 mins, or till the chicken is fully cooked, and the stuffing is hot and bubbly. Take out from the oven and let the chicken rest for a couple of mins before presenting.

Nutritional Info: Calories: 305, Fat: 16g, Carbohydrates: 3g, Protein: 34g

3. Greek-inspired Cucumber and Tomato Salad

(Setup Time: 15 mins | How Many People: 4)

Rich in antioxidants, vitamins, and minerals, such as vitamin C, potassium, and calcium, this salad provides seniors with a nourishing meal that supports immune function and bone health.

Additionally, the heart-healthy fats found in olive oil and olives contribute to satiety and promote overall well-being.

Recipe Components:

- 4 medium-sized cucumbers, skinned and carved
- 4 big tomatoes, cubed
- 1/2 red onion, finely cut
- 1 teacup Kalamata olives, pitted and halved
- 1 teacup crumbled feta cheese
- 1/4 teacup fresh parsley, severed
- 1/4 teacup fresh mint, severed

Dressing Ingredients:

- 1/4 teacup extra-virgin olive oil
- 2 tbsps red wine vinegar
- 2 pieces garlic, crushed
- 1 tsp dried oregano
- Salt and pepper as required

Preparation Steps: Inside a big salad container, blend the carved cucumbers, cubed tomatoes, carved red onion, Kalamata olives, crumbled feta cheese, severed parsley, and severed mint. Inside a distinct small container, whisk collectively the olive oil, red wine vinegar, crushed garlic, dried oregano, salt, and pepper to make the dressing. Pour the dressing over the salad components in the big container. Shake the salad gently to ensure that all components are well covered with the dressing. Allow the salad to relax for around 10 mins to allow the flavors to meld together. Serve the Greek-inspired Cucumber and Tomato Salad as a refreshing side dish or a light main course.

Nutritional Info: Calories: 285, Fat: 23g, Carb: 15g, Protein: 6g

4. Zucchini Noodles with Pesto and Cherry Tomatoes

(Setup Time: 15 mins | Cooked in: 15 mins | How Many People: 4)

Low in carbohydrates and rich in fiber, vitamins, and minerals, such as vitamin C, potassium, and antioxidants, this dish provides seniors with a nourishing meal that supports digestive health and immune function. Additionally, the healthy fats found in olive oil and pesto contribute to satiety and help maintain stable blood sugar levels. Light yet satisfying, our Zucchini Noodles with Pesto and Cherry Tomatoes offer seniors a delicious lunch option that's both nutritious and delicious.

Recipe Components:

- 4 medium zucchinis
- 1 pint cherry tomatoes
- 1/2 teacup basil pesto

- 1/4 teacup grated Parmesan cheese
- Salt and pepper as required
- Red pepper flakes (optional, for heat)

Preparation Steps: Using a spiralizer, make zucchini noodles from the zucchinis. Put away. Inside a big pan, warm olive oil at med temp. Include cherry tomatoes and cook for 2-3 mins till they start to blister. Include the zucchini noodles to the pan, and cook for an extra 2-3 mins till they are mildly soft. Stir in the basil pesto and cook for an extra 2 mins, ensuring the noodles are well covered. Season with salt and pepper as required.

If you like it spicy, include red pepper flakes. Serve hot, garnished with grated Parmesan cheese.

Nutritional Info: Calories: 220, Fat: 17g, Carb: 10g, Protein: 8g, Fiber: 3g

5. Keto Beef and Broccoli

(Setup Time: 10 mins | Cooked in: 20 mins | How Many People: 4)

This savory Asian dish features tender slices of beef sirloin stir-fried with crisp broccoli florets in a rich and flavorful sauce made with soy sauce, sesame oil, garlic, and ginger. High in protein and packed with essential nutrients, such as iron, vitamin C, and fiber, this dish provides seniors with a nourishing meal that supports muscle health and digestive function. Moreover, the inclusion of broccoli adds a nutritional boost, providing antioxidants and phytonutrients that promote overall well-being.

Recipe Components:

- 1 lb. of beef sirloin, finely cut
- 4 teacups of broccoli florets
- 3 pieces of garlic, crushed
- 1/4 teacup of soy sauce (or coconut aminos for a gluten-free option)
- 2 tbsps of olive oil
- 1 tbsp of sesame oil
- 1 tbsp of erythritol or your preferred keto-friendly sweetener
- 1/2 tsp of ginger, crushed
- 1/2 tsp of xanthan gum (for densesing)
- Salt and pepper as required
- Sesame seeds and carved green onions for garnish (optional)

Preparation Steps: Inside a big griddle or wok, warm olive oil at med-high temp. Include the beef slices and cook for 2-3 mins or till browned. Take out the beef from the griddle and put it away. Inside the same griddle, include garlic and ginger. Sauté for around 30 secs. Include broccoli florets and sauté for 3-4 mins till they start to become soft. Inside a container, mix soy sauce, sesame oil, erythritol, and xanthan gum. Stir till thoroughly mixed. Return the beef to the griddle and pour the sauce over the beef and broccoli. Cook for an extra 2-3 mins till the sauce densess. Season with salt and pepper as required. Garnish with sesame seeds and carved green onions, if wanted.

Nutritional Info: Calories: 290, Fat: 20g, Carb: 7g, Fiber: 2g, Protein: 23g

6. Baked Cod with Lemon and Dill

(Setup Time: 10 mins | Cooked in: 20 mins | How Many People: 4)

Rich in protein and heart-healthy fats, such as omega-3 fatty acids, cod is an excellent source of nutrients that support cognitive function, cardiovascular health, and muscle maintenance in seniors. Moreover, the addition of lemon and dill not only enhances the taste but also provides a refreshing burst of vitamin C and antioxidants, which promote immune function and overall well-being.

Recipe Components:

- 4 cod fillets
- 2 tbsps of olive oil
- 2 pieces of garlic, crushed
- 1 lemon, finely cut
- 1/4 teacup of fresh dill, severed
- Salt and pepper as required
- Lemon wedges for presenting

Preparation Steps: Warm up your oven to 375 deg.F (190 deg.C). Grease a baking dish with olive oil. Put the cod fillets in the baking dish. Spray the olive oil over the fillets and season them with crushed garlic, salt, and pepper. Lay lemon slices on top of the cod fillets. Spray fresh dill over the fillets and lemon slices. Cover the baking dish with foil and bake for 15 mins. Take out the foil and bake for an extra 5 mins or till the cod is flaky and fully cooked. Serve with lemon wedges.

Nutritional Info: Calories: 220, Fat: 8g, Carb: 2g, Protein: 34g

7. Asparagus and Prosciutto Wraps

(Setup Time: 15 mins | Cooked in: 12 mins | How Many People: 4)

Low in carbohydrates and rich in essential nutrients, such as vitamin K, folate, and fiber, asparagus is a nutritional powerhouse that supports digestive health, bone strength, and immune function in seniors. Additionally, prosciutto adds a flavorful punch while providing high-quality protein and healthy fats, making it an ideal choice for seniors looking to maintain muscle mass and overall well-being.

Recipe Components:

- 12 fresh asparagus spears
- 6 slices of prosciutto
- 1 tbsp olive oil
- Salt and pepper as required
- Balsamic vinegar for drizzling (optional)

Preparation Steps: Warm up your oven to 400 deg.F (200 deg.C). Trim the tough ends of the asparagus. Take two asparagus spears and wrap them in one slice of prosciutto, repeat for the entire asparagus. Put the prosciutto-wrapped asparagus on a baking sheet. Spray olive oil over the asparagus and season with salt and pepper. Roast in the warmed up oven for 10-12 mins or till the asparagus is soft and the prosciutto is crispy. Optionally, spray with balsamic vinegar before presenting.

Nutritional Info: Calories: 90, Fat: 6g, Carb: 2g, Protein: 7g

8. Eggplant Parmesan

(Setup Time: 30 mins | Cooked in: 40 mins | How Many People: 6)

This mouthwatering dish features tender eggplant slices coated in a crispy breadcrumb mixture, fried to golden perfection, and layered with rich marinara sauce, gooey mozzarella cheese, and savory Parmesan cheese. Eggplant, the star ingredient of this dish, is not only low in carbs but also rich in fiber, antioxidants, and vitamins, making it an excellent choice for seniors looking to maintain a healthy weight and support overall well-being.

Moreover, the addition of marinara sauce provides a burst of flavor and essential nutrients, while mozzarella and Parmesan cheese add a creamy richness that's simply irresistible.

Recipe Components:

- 2 big eggplants
- 2 teacups marinara sauce
- 2 teacups mozzarella cheese, shredded
- 1/2 teacup Parmesan cheese, grated
- 2 teacups all-purpose flour
- 3 big eggs

- 2 teacups breadcrumbs
- 2 tsps dried basil
- 2 tsps dried oregano
- Salt and pepper as required
- Olive oil for frying
- Fresh basil leaves for garnish (optional)

Preparation Steps: Slice the eggplants into 1/2-inch dense rounds. Inside a container, mix breadcrumbs with dried basil, dried oregano, salt, and pepper. Dredge each eggplant slice in flour, then dip into beaten eggs, and cover with the breadcrumb mixture. Inside a big griddle, warm olive oil at med-high temp. Fry the eggplant slices till golden brown. Put them on paper towels to drain excess oil. Warm up the oven to 375 deg.F (190 deg.C). Inside a baking dish, spread a fine layer of marinara sauce. Put a layer of fried eggplant slices, followed by mozzarella and Parmesan cheese. Repeat the layers. Bake in the warmed up oven for 25-30 mins or till the cheese is bubbly and golden. Garnish with fresh basil leaves if wanted.

Nutritional Info: Calories: 420, Fat: 19g, Carb: 45g, Protein: 18g

9. Shrimp and Cauliflower Rice Stir-Fry

(Setup Time: 10 mins | Cooked in: 15 mins | How Many People: 4)

This delightful dish features succulent shrimp, tender cauliflower rice, and a colorful array of vegetables stir-fried to perfection in a fragrant blend of garlic, ginger, and soy sauce. Bursting with protein, fiber, and essential nutrients, each bite offers a satisfying combination of flavors and textures that's sure to delight your senses and leave you feeling nourished and satisfied. Shrimp, a lean source of protein, is not only low in carbs but also rich in omega-3 fatty acids, which support heart health and cognitive function in seniors. Additionally, cauliflower rice serves as a nutritious alternative to traditional rice, providing a low-carb, high-fiber option that's perfect for those following a ketogenic diet.

Recipe Components:

- 1 lb. of shrimp, skinned and deveined
- 4 teacups of cauliflower rice
- 2 tbsps of oil (e.g., olive oil or sesame oil)
- Vegetables of your choice (e.g., bell peppers, broccoli, carrots)
- Sauce components (e.g., soy sauce, garlic, ginger, and optional chili flakes)
- Optional garnishes (e.g., green onions and sesame seeds)

Preparation Steps: Heat oil in a big griddle or wok at med-high temp. Include garlic and ginger, stir for around 30 secs. Include shrimp and stir-fry till they turn pink and opaque. Take out the shrimp from the griddle. Inside the same griddle, include more oil if needed and stir-fry your choice of vegetables till they are soft-crisp. Include cauliflower rice and cook for a couple of mins till it's fully heated. Return the shrimp to the griddle. Include the sauce components and stir-fry for a couple of mins till everything is thoroughly mixed and heated. Serve hot, garnished with green onions and sesame seeds if wanted.

Nutritional Info: Calories: 250-300 kcal, Protein: 25-30g, Carb: 10-15g, Fat: 10-15g

10. Cauliflower and Bacon Soup

(Setup Time: 15 mins | Cooked in: 35 mins | How Many People: 4)

Cauliflower takes center stage in this recipe, offering a low-carb alternative packed with essential vitamins, minerals, and antioxidants to support overall health and well-being in seniors. Meanwhile, bacon lends its savory essence, providing a satisfying dose of protein and healthy fats that contribute to a balanced ketogenic meal.

Recipe Components:

- 1 medium-sized cauliflower head, cut into florets
- 4-6 slices of bacon, severed
- 1 onion, finely severed
- 2 pieces of garlic, crushed
- 4 teacups chicken or vegetable broth
- 1 teacup heavy cream
- Salt and pepper as required
- Chopped fresh chives for garnish (optional)

Preparation Steps: Inside a big soup pot, cook the severed bacon at med temp. till it's crispy. Take out some of the bacon bits for garnish, leaving some in the pot for flavor. Include the severed onion to the pot and cook till it's translucent. Stir in the crushed garlic and cook for an extra min. Include the cauliflower florets and sauté for a couple of mins. Pour in the chicken or vegetable broth and bring the mixture to a boil. Reduce the heat and simmer till the cauliflower is soft. Make the soup as smooth as possible by blending it with an immersion mixer. If you lack access to an immersion mixer, you may move the soup to a regular mixer in stages and puree it till it's smooth. After that, you can put it back in the pot. Stir in the heavy cream and season with salt and pepper as required. Serve hot, garnished with the reserved crispy bacon bits and severed chives if wanted.

Nutritional Info: Calories: 300-350 kcal, Protein: 8-10g, Carb: 10-15g, Fat: 20-25g

11. Avocado and Tuna Stuffed Bell Peppers

(Setup Time: 20 mins | How Many People: 2)

These bell peppers are not only bursting with flavor but also offer a host of benefits for older adults. The creamy avocado and protein-rich tuna provide essential nutrients and healthy fats, supporting brain health and providing sustained energy throughout the day.

The addition of red onion and cucumber adds a refreshing crunch and extra vitamins and minerals, contributing to overall well-being.

Recipe Components:

- 2 big bell peppers (any color)
- 1 can (5 oz) of canned tuna, drained
- 1 ripe avocado, cubed
- 1/4 teacup red onion, finely severed
- 1/4 teacup cucumber, cubed
- 2 tbsps mayonnaise
- 1 tbsp lemon juice
- Salt and pepper as required
- Fresh parsley or cilantro for garnish (optional)

Preparation Steps: Cut the tops off the bell peppers and take out the seeds and membranes. Put them away. Inside a blending container, blend the drained canned tuna, cubed avocado, severed red onion, cubed cucumber, mayonnaise, and lemon juice. Mix everything together. Season the mixture with salt and pepper as required. Stuff each bell pepper with the tuna and avocado mixture, pressing it down gently to fill the peppers. Garnish with fresh parsley or cilantro if wanted. Serve instantly, or put in the fridge till ready to serve.

Nutritional Info: Calories: 300-350 kcal, Protein: 15-20g, Carb: 10-15g, Fat: 20-25g

12. Keto Turkey and Cranberry Salad

(Setup Time: 10 mins | How Many People: 2)

This salad offers a perfect blend of protein, healthy fats, and low-carb ingredients, making it an excellent choice for older adults following a ketogenic lifestyle. The tender cubes of turkey breast provide a lean source of protein, supporting muscle health and satiety. Fresh cranberries add a tangy burst of flavor and antioxidants, promoting immune function and overall vitality. Pecans or walnuts offer healthy fats and crunchy texture, while celery adds fiber and essential vitamins.

Recipe Components:

- 2 teacups of cooked turkey breast, cubed
- 1/2 teacup of fresh cranberries, halved
- 1/4 teacup of severed pecans or walnuts
- 1/4 teacup of cubed celery
- 2 tbsps of mayonnaise
- 1 tbsp of Greek yogurt (optional)
- 1 tbsp of fresh lemon juice
- Salt and pepper as required
- Lettuce leaves for presenting (optional)

Preparation Steps: Inside a blending container, blend the cubed turkey breast, halved cranberries, severed nuts, and cubed celery. Inside a separate small container, mix the mayonnaise, Greek yogurt (if using), and fresh lemon juice. This will be your dressing. Pour the dressing over the turkey and cranberry mixture and shake till everything is well covered. Season with salt and pepper as required. If desired, serve the salad on a bed of lettuce leaves.

Nutritional Info: Calories: 300-350 kcal, Protein: 25-30g, Carb: 5-10g, Fat: 15-20g

13. Keto Cabbage Rolls

(Setup Time: 20 mins | Cooked in: 45-60 mins | How Many People: 4)

These hearty rolls offer a comforting and satisfying meal without compromising on flavor or nutritional value. The combination of ground beef or turkey, cauliflower rice, and aromatic seasonings provides a delicious and filling filling that's low in carbs and high in protein, making it an ideal choice for older adults following a keto lifestyle. The addition of cabbage leaves adds fiber and essential nutrients, promoting digestive health and satiety. With just 300-350 calories per serving and a balanced macronutrient profile, including moderate protein and low carbohydrates, these cabbage rolls are a nourishing and satisfying option for seniors looking to maintain ketosis while enjoying a classic comfort food dish.

Recipe Components:

- 8 big cabbage leaves
- 1 lb. ground beef or ground turkey
- 1/2 teacup cauliflower rice
- 1/4 teacup cubed onion
- 1 piece garlic, crushed
- 1/4 teacup cubed tomatoes
- 1 tsp Italian seasoning
- Salt and pepper as required
- 1 teacup sugar-free tomato sauce
- 1/2 teacup beef or vegetable broth
- Shredded mozzarella cheese (optional)
- Chopped fresh parsley for garnish

Preparation Steps: Bring a big pot of water to a boil. Carefully blanch the cabbage leaves for around 2-3 mins till they are pliable. Drain and put away. Inside a griddle, brown the ground beef or turkey at med temp. Include cubed onion and garlic. Cook till the meat is no longer pink and the onion is translucent. Stir in the cauliflower rice, cubed tomatoes, Italian seasoning, salt, and pepper. Cook for an extra 5 mins. Warm up the oven to 350 deg.F (175 deg.C). Put a portion of the meat mixture in the center of each cabbage leaf. Roll them up, tucking in the sides to create rolls. Inside a baking dish, spread some tomato sauce on the bottom. Put the cabbage rolls in the dish. Pour the rest of the tomato sauce and broth over the cabbage rolls. Spray with mozzarella cheese if wanted. Cover with foil and bake for 45-60 mins till the cabbage is soft. Garnish with severed parsley before presenting.

Nutritional Info: Calories: 300-350 kcal, Protein: 20-25g, Carb: 10-15g, Fat: 10-15g

14. Thai Coconut Chicken Soup

(Setup Time: 10 mins | Cooked in: 20-25 mins | How Many People: 4)

Transport your taste buds to Thailand with the Thai Coconut Chicken Soup, perfect for seniors seeking a flavorful and nourishing meal on the ketogenic diet. This aromatic soup is rich in protein, healthy fats, and low in carbohydrates, making it an ideal option for older adults looking to support their health goals. The tender chicken breast, simmered in a creamy coconut milk broth infused with aromatic spices and fresh vegetables, provides a comforting and satisfying meal that's both delicious and nutritious. The addition of mushrooms, tomatoes, and onions adds vitamins, minerals, and antioxidants, supporting immune function and overall well-being.

Recipe Components:

- 1 lb. boneless, skinless chicken breasts, finely cut
- 1 can (14 oz.) coconut milk
- 4 teacups chicken broth
- 1 stalk lemongrass, cut into 2-inch pieces and smashed
- 3-4 slices galangal or ginger
- 2-3 kaffir lime leaves, torn into pieces
- 2-3 red bird's eye chilies, smashed (adjust to your preferred level of spiciness)

- 200g (about 7 oz.) white mushrooms, carved
- 1 medium tomato, cut into wedges
- 1 small onion, finely cut
- 2-3 pieces garlic, crushed
- 2-3 tbsps fish sauce (adjust as required)
- 1-2 tbsps lime juice (adjust as required)
- 1 tsp brown sugar (optional)
- Fresh cilantro leaves and carved red chilies for garnish

Preparation Steps: Inside a pot, bring the chicken broth to a boil. Include the lemongrass, galangal or ginger, kaffir lime leaves, and smashed red chilies. Simmer for around 10 mins to infuse the flavors. Include the carved chicken to the pot and simmer till it's no longer pink, around 5-7 mins. Stir in the coconut milk and let it simmer for an extra 2-3 mins. Include the mushrooms, tomato, onion, and garlic. Cook till the vegetables are soft, around 3-4 mins. Season the soup with fish sauce, lime juice, and brown sugar (if using). Adjust the seasonings to your taste. Take out the lemongrass, galangal or ginger, kaffir lime leaves, and smashed red chilies. Serve the soup hot, garnished with fresh cilantro leaves and carved red chilies.

Nutritional Info: Calories: 250-300 kcal, Protein: 25-30g, Carb: 6-8g, Fat: 15-18g

15. Spinach and Mushroom Stuffed Pork Chops

(Setup Time: 15 mins | Cooked in: 30-35 mins | How Many People: 4)

These succulent pork chops offer a delightful combination of flavors and textures, making them a favorite among older adults seeking a satisfying and nutritious meal. The savory filling, made with sautéed mushrooms, spinach, garlic, and onions, provides a rich source of vitamins, minerals, and antioxidants, supporting overall health and well-being.

The addition of breadcrumbs and Parmesan cheese adds a crunchy texture and extra flavor without compromising on nutritional value.

Recipe Components:

- 4 bone-in pork chops
- 1 teacup baby spinach, severed
- 1 teacup mushrooms, finely severed
- 1/2 teacup breadcrumbs
- 1/4 teacup Parmesan cheese, grated
- 2 pieces garlic, crushed
- 1/4 teacup onion, finely severed
- 1 egg
- 2 tbsps olive oil
- Salt and pepper as required
- Cooking twine (optional)

Preparation Steps: Warm up your oven to 375 deg.F (190 deg.C). Inside a griddle, heat 1 tbsp of olive oil at med temp. Include the garlic and onions and sauté till they become translucent, around 2-3 mins. Include the severed mushrooms and cook till they release their moisture and become soft, around 5-7 mins. Season with salt and pepper. Take out from heat and let it cool. Inside a blending container, blend the sautéed mushroom mixture with the severed baby spinach, breadcrumbs, grated Parmesan cheese, and the egg. Mix till all components are thoroughly mixed. Carefully cut a pocket into each pork chop without cutting the entire way through. Stuff each pork chop with the spinach and mushroom mixture. If desired, use cooking twine to secure the stuffed pork chops. Heat the rest of the 1 tbsp of olive oil in an oven-safe griddle at med-high temp. Brown the stuffed pork chops on both sides for around 2-3 mins on all sides. Transfer the griddle to the warmed up oven and bake for 20-25 mins, or till the pork reaches an internal temp. of 145 deg.F (63 deg.C) and the stuffing is golden brown. Let the stuffed pork chops rest for a couple of mins before presenting.

Nutritional Info: Calories: 300-350 kcal, Protein: 30-35g, Carb: 10-15g, Fat: 15-18g

16. Creamy Garlic Shrimp with Spinach

(Setup Time: 10 mins | Cooked in: 15-20 mins | How Many People: 4)

Featuring succulent shrimp cooked to perfection in a buttery garlic sauce, paired with vibrant cherry tomatoes and nutrient-rich spinach, this dish offers a satisfying combination of flavors and textures. The addition of heavy cream and grated Parmesan cheese creates a luxurious creamy sauce that is both comforting and delicious. With just 300-350 calories per serving and a balanced macronutrient profile of 25-30g of protein, 6-8g of carbs, and 20-25g of healthy fats, our Creamy Garlic Shrimp with Spinach provides seniors with a nourishing meal that supports their dietary goals while satisfying their taste buds. Garnish with fresh basil leaves for a touch of brightness and serve alongside your favorite low-carb sides for a complete and satisfying meal.

Recipe Components:

- 1 lb. big shrimp, skinned and deveined
- 2 tbsps butter
- 4 pieces garlic, crushed
- 1 teacup cherry tomatoes, halved
- 4 teacups fresh spinach

- 1 teacup heavy cream
- 1/4 teacup grated Parmesan cheese
- Salt and pepper as required
- Fresh basil leaves for garnish (optional)

Preparation Steps: Inside a big griddle, dissolve the butter at med-high temp. Include the crushed garlic and sauté for around 1 min, till fragrant. Include the shrimp to the griddle and cook for 2-3 mins on all sides or till they turn pink and opaque. Take out the cooked shrimp from the griddle and put away. Inside the same griddle, include the halved cherry tomatoes and cook for around 2 mins till they start to soften. Stir in the fresh spinach and cook till it wilts, around 2-3 mins. Pour in the heavy cream and grated Parmesan cheese. Stir well to blend and let it simmer for 2-3 mins, allowing the sauce to denses. Return the cooked shrimp to the griddle and heat through for an extra 2 mins.

Season with salt and pepper as required. Garnish with fresh basil leaves if wanted.

Nutritional Info: Calories: 300-350 kcal, Protein: 25-30g, Carb: 6-8g, Fat: 20-25g

17. Greek Lemon Chicken Soup (Avgolemono Soup)
(Setup Time: 10 mins | Cooked in: 25-30 mins | How Many People: 4)

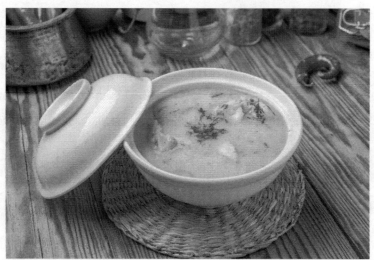

The soup features chicken broth, shredded chicken, and orzo pasta, providing protein and essential nutrients while keeping the carb content in check. The addition of eggs, lemon juice, and zest not only enhances the flavor but also adds a creamy texture without relying on high-carb thickeners. With a moderate amount of protein and low-carb content, this soup is ideal for seniors looking to maintain ketosis while enjoying a taste of Greek cuisine.

Recipe Components:

- 4 teacups chicken broth
- 2 boneless, skinless chicken breasts, cooked and shredded
- 1/2 teacup orzo pasta
- 2 big eggs
- Juice of 2 lemons
- Zest of 1 lemon
- Salt and pepper as required
- Fresh dill for garnish (optional)

Preparation Steps: Inside a big pot, bring the chicken broth to a boil. Include the orzo pasta and cook as per to the package guidelines till al dente. Once the orzo is cooked, include the shredded chicken to the pot. Let it simmer for a couple of mins. Inside a distinct container, whisk collectively the eggs, lemon juice, and lemon zest till thoroughly mixed. While continuously whisking, slowly pour a ladleful of the hot broth into the egg-lemon mixture. This tempers the eggs and prevents them from curdling. Slowly pour the egg-lemon mixture back into the pot with the soup, mixing regularly. Keep the heat low to avoid curdling. Continue to cook for a couple of more mins till the soup densess mildly. Season with salt and pepper as required. Garnish with fresh dill, if wanted.

Nutritional Info: Calories: 250-300 kcal, Protein: 20-25g, Carb: 20-25g, Fat: 5-7g

18. Keto BLT Salad

(Setup Time: 10 mins | Cooked in: 5 mins | How Many People: 4)

This keto BLT salad is a refreshing and satisfying option for seniors following a ketogenic diet. With a setup time of just 10 minutes and cooked in around 5 minutes, it's quick and easy to prepare, making it suitable for seniors who prefer simple and hassle-free meals. The salad features crisp romaine lettuce, juicy cherry tomatoes, and savory bacon crumbles, providing a variety of textures and flavors. The creamy dressing, made with mayonnaise, sour cream, and Dijon mustard, adds richness and tanginess without compromising on the ketogenic principles. With a balanced ratio of protein, fat, and low-carb content, this salad is a delicious choice for seniors looking to maintain ketosis while enjoying a classic BLT flavor.

Recipe Components:

- 6 teacups severed romaine lettuce
- 1 teacup cherry tomatoes, halved
- 1/2 teacup cooked and crumbled bacon
- 1/4 teacup mayonnaise
- 2 tbsps sour cream
- 1 tsp Dijon mustard
- Salt and pepper as required
- Optional: grated Parmesan cheese

Preparation Steps: Inside a big salad containers, blend the severed romaine lettuce, halved cherry tomatoes, and crumbled bacon. Inside a distinct small container, whisk collectively the mayonnaise, sour cream, and Dijon mustard till thoroughly mixed. Season the dressing with salt and pepper as required. Pour the dressing over the salad and shake to cover the components evenly. Top the salad with grated Parmesan cheese if wanted.

Nutritional Info: Calories: 250-300 kcal, Protein: 5-7g, Carb: 5-7g, Fat: 20-25g

19. Spinach and Artichoke Stuffed Chicken

(Setup Time: 15 mins | Cooked in: 30-35 mins | How Many People: 4)

This dish features tender chicken breasts stuffed with a mixture of spinach, artichoke hearts, cream cheese, and Parmesan cheese, offering a delicious combination of textures and flavors. With a moderate amount of protein and low-carb content, this dish is suitable for seniors looking to maintain ketosis while enjoying a satisfying and filling meal.

Recipe Components:

- 4 boneless, skinless chicken breasts
- 1 teacup frozen severed spinach, thawed and drained
- 1 teacup canned artichoke hearts, drained and severed
- 1/2 teacup cream cheese
- 1/4 teacup grated Parmesan cheese
- 2 pieces garlic, crushed
- Salt and pepper as required
- Olive oil for cooking
- Optional: additional grated Parmesan for toppinge

Preparation Steps: Warm up your oven to 375 deg.F (190 deg.C). Inside a blending container, blend the severed spinach, severed artichoke hearts, cream cheese, grated Parmesan, crushed garlic, and season with salt and pepper. Carefully butterfly each chicken breast by slicing horizontally through the center but not the entire way through, creating a pocket. Stuff each chicken breast with the spinach and artichoke mixture. Warm olive oil in an ovenproof griddle at med-high temp. Put the stuffed chicken breasts in the griddle and cook for 3-4 mins on all sides till they are nicely browned. Transfer the griddle to the warmed up oven and bake for 20-25 mins or till the chicken is fully cooked. Optional: Spray additional grated Parmesan on top of each chicken breast during the last 5 mins of baking. Take out from the oven, allow it to relax for a couple of mins, and serve.

Nutritional Info: Calories: 300-350 kcal, Protein: 30-35g, Carb: 5-7g, Fat: 15-20g

20. Salmon and Avocado Salad

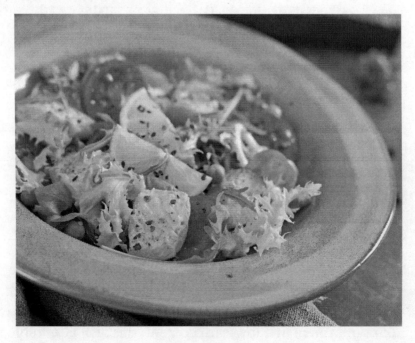

(Setup Time: 15 mins | Cooked in: 10-15 mins | How Many People: 2)

This salmon and avocado salad is a light yet satisfying option for seniors following a ketogenic diet. With a setup time of just 15 minutes and cooked in around 10-15 minutes, it's quick and easy to prepare, perfect for seniors who prefer meals that are both nutritious and effortless. The salad features grilled salmon fillets served atop a bed of mixed greens, avocado, cherry tomatoes, and cucumber, providing a variety of flavors and nutrients. The balsamic vinaigrette dressing adds a tangy and refreshing touch without adding unnecessary carbs. With a balanced ratio of protein, healthy fats, and low-carb content, this salad is an excellent choice for seniors looking to maintain ketosis while enjoying a delicious and wholesome meal.

Recipe Components:

- 2 salmon fillets (about 6-8 oz. each)
- 2 tbsps olive oil
- Salt and pepper as required
- 4 teacups mixed salad greens (e.g., lettuce, spinach, arugula)
- 1 avocado, carved
- 1/2 red onion, finely cut
- 1/2 teacup cherry tomatoes, halved
- 1/4 teacup cucumber, carved
- 2 tbsps balsamic vinaigrette dressing
- Optional: lemon wedges for garnish

Preparation Steps: Warm up your grill or a grill pan to med-high temp. Brush the salmon fillets with olive oil and season with salt and pepper. Put the salmon fillets on the grill and cook for around 4-5 mins on all sides, or till the salmon is cooked to your desired level of doneness. While the salmon is cooking, prepare your salad. Inside a big container, blend the mixed salad greens, carved avocado, red onion, cherry tomatoes, and cucumber. Once the salmon is done, take out it from the grill and allow it to relax for a couple of mins. To assemble the salad, place a generous portion of the salad mixture on each plate. Top the salad with a grilled salmon fillet. Spray the balsamic vinaigrette dressing over the salad.

Optional: Garnish with lemon wedges for added flavor.

Nutritional Info: Calories: 400-450 kcal, Protein: 30-35g, Carb: 10-15g, Fat: 25-30g

Chapter 8: Keto Recipes For Dinner

1. Creamy Spinach and Mushroom Stuffed Pork Tenderloin
(Setup Time: 15 mins | Cooked in: 40 mins | How Many People: 4)

Ideal for seniors following a ketogenic diet, this dish offers a flavorful and nutrient-rich option. The tender pork tenderloin is stuffed with a creamy mixture of spinach and mushrooms, providing essential vitamins and minerals. With setup and cooking times kept to a minimum, it's a convenient choice for a satisfying dinner.

Recipe Components:

- 1 pork tenderloin (about 1 lb.)
- 1 teacup of fresh spinach, severed
- 1 teacup of mushrooms, finely severed
- 2 pieces of garlic, crushed
- 1/2 teacup of cream cheese
- 1/4 teacup of grated Parmesan cheese
- 1 tbsp of olive oil
- Salt and pepper as required
- Kitchen twine for tying the pork

Preparation Steps: Warm up your oven to 375 deg.F (190 deg.C). Inside a griddle, warm olive oil at med temp. Include crushed garlic and sauté for around 1 min till fragrant. Include severed mushrooms to the griddle and cook till they release their moisture and become soft, around 5 mins. Season with salt and pepper. Stir in the severed spinach and cook for an extra 2 mins till it wilts. Take out the griddle from heat. Inside a container, blend the sautéed mushroom and spinach mixture with cream cheese and grated Parmesan. Mix well till you have a creamy filling. Butterfly the pork tenderloin by making a lengthwise cut down the center, without cutting the entire way through, and then open it up like a book. Spread the creamy spinach and mushroom mixture evenly over the inside of the pork tenderloin. Roll the stuffed pork tenderloin and secure it with kitchen twine at 1-inch intervals. Put the stuffed pork tenderloin in a baking dish and season the outside with salt and pepper. Roast in the warmed up oven for around 30-35 mins or till the internal temp. reaches 145 deg.F (63 deg.C). Take out from the oven and allow it to relax for a couple of mins before slicing. Slice the stuffed pork tenderloin, serve, and enjoy!

Nutritional Info: Calories: 300 kcal, Protein: 30g, Carb: 4g, Fat: 18g

2. Keto Eggplant Lasagna
(Setup Time: 20 mins | Cooked in: 45 mins | How Many People: 6)

This keto-friendly eggplant lasagna is perfect for seniors looking for a low-carb alternative to traditional lasagna. By replacing noodles with thinly sliced eggplant, it reduces carb intake while still offering the comforting flavors of a classic dish. With ample protein and healthy fats from the cheeses and meats, it's a filling and nutritious option.

Recipe Components:

- 1 big eggplant, finely cut lengthwise
- 1 lb. ground beef (or ground turkey for a leaner option)
- 1/2 teacup cubed onions
- 2 pieces garlic, crushed
- 1 1/2 teacups marinara sauce (look for a low-carb version)
- 1 teacup ricotta cheese
- 1 teacup shredded mozzarella cheese
- 1/4 teacup grated Parmesan cheese
- 2 tbsps olive oil
- 1 tsp dried basil
- 1 tsp dried oregano
- Salt and pepper as required
- Fresh basil leaves for garnish (optional)

Preparation Steps: Warm up your oven to 375 deg.F (190 deg.C). Lay the carved eggplant on a baking sheet, spray with olive oil, and season with salt and pepper. Roast in the oven for around 15-20 mins or till soft. Take out and put away. Inside a griddle, warm olive oil at med temp. Include cubed onions and cook till they become translucent, around 2-3 mins. Include crushed garlic and sauté for an extra min. Include ground beef (or turkey) to the griddle and cook till browned and fully cooked. Drain any excess fat. Stir in the marinara sauce, dried basil, and dried oregano. Let it simmer for a couple of mins. Inside a distinct container, mix the ricotta cheese with a tweak of salt and pepper. Inside a baking dish, start assembling the lasagna. Begin with a layer of roasted eggplant slices, followed by a layer of the meat sauce, a layer of ricotta cheese, and a layer of mozzarella cheese. Repeat till all components are utilized. Top the lasagna with the grated Parmesan cheese. Bake in the warmed up oven for around 20-25 mins, or till the cheese is bubbly and golden. Let it cool for a couple of mins, garnish with fresh basil leaves (if wanted), slice, and serve.

Nutritional Info: Calories: 350 kcal, Protein: 25g, Carb: 9g, Fat: 24g

3. Dijon and Herb Crusted Salmon

(Setup Time: 10 mins | Cooked in: 15 mins | How Many People: 4)

Rich in omega-3 fatty acids and protein, salmon is an excellent choice for seniors on a ketogenic diet. This recipe adds a flavorful twist with a Dijon and herb crust, providing a satisfying crunch without added carbs. With minimal prep and cook time, it's a quick and easy option for a nutritious dinner.

Recipe Components:

- 4 salmon fillets
- 2 tbsps Dijon mustard
- 1/4 teacup fresh breadcrumbs (or almond flour for a low-carb option)
- 2 tbsps fresh parsley, severed
- 1 tbsp fresh dill, severed
- 2 pieces garlic, crushed
- 2 tbsps olive oil
- Salt and pepper as required
- Lemon wedges for garnish

Preparation Steps: Warm up your oven to 400 deg.F (200 deg.C). Inside a small container, blend the Dijon mustard, fresh breadcrumbs (or almond flour), fresh parsley, fresh dill, crushed garlic, olive oil, salt, and pepper. Mix well to form a crumbly mixture. Put the salmon fillets on a baking sheet lined with parchment paper. Spread the Dijon and herb mixture evenly over the top of each salmon fillet, pressing it down gently to adhere. Bake in the warmed up oven for around 12-15 mins or till the salmon flakes simply with a fork and the crust is golden. Take out from the oven, garnish with lemon wedges, and serve hot.

Nutritional Info: Cal: 300 kcal, Protein: 25g, Carb: 5g (or lower with almond flour), Fat: 20g

4. Keto Beef Stroganoff

(Setup Time: 10 mins | Cooked in: 20 mins | How Many People: 4)

Seniors will appreciate the tender beef and creamy sauce in this keto beef stroganoff, which is served over cauliflower rice or zucchini noodles for a low-carb option. With plenty of protein and healthy fats from the beef and sour cream, it's a comforting and satisfying meal that's easy to digest.

Recipe Components:

- 1 lb. of beef sirloin or tenderloin, finely cut
- 2 tbsps of butter
- 1 small onion, finely severed
- 2 pieces of garlic, crushed
- 8 oz. of mushrooms, carved
- 1 teacup of beef broth

- 1/2 teacup of sour cream
- 1 tbsp of Dijon mustard
- 1 tbsp of Worcestershire sauce
- Salt and pepper as required
- Fresh parsley, severed, for garnish
- Cauliflower rice or zucchini noodles for presenting

Preparation Steps: Inside a big griddle, dissolve the butter at med temp. Include the severed onion and garlic, and sauté till they become translucent. Include the finely cut beef to the griddle and cook for a couple of mins till it's browned on all sides. Take out the beef from the griddle and put it away. Inside the same griddle, include the carved mushrooms and cook till they release their moisture and become soft. Return the cooked beef to the griddle with the mushrooms. Stir in the beef broth, sour cream, Dijon mustard, and Worcestershire sauce. Simmer the mixture for around 5-7 mins, allowing the flavors to meld and the sauce to denses. Season with salt and pepper as required. Serve the Keto Beef Stroganoff over cauliflower rice or zucchini noodles. Garnish with severed fresh parsley before presenting.

Nutritional Info: Calories: 350 kcal, Protein: 30g, Carb: 5g, Fat: 22g

5. Lemon Garlic Shrimp and Zucchini Noodles

(Setup Time: 15 mins | Cooked in: 10 mins | How Many People: 2)

For a light and refreshing option, this lemon garlic shrimp with zucchini noodles is a perfect choice. The shrimp provides protein while the zucchini noodles offer a low-carb alternative to traditional pasta.

With a burst of citrus flavor from lemon and garlic, it's a flavorful dish that's quick to prepare and full of essential nutrients.

Recipe Components:

- 8 oz. of big shrimp, skinned and deveined
- 2 medium-sized zucchinis
- 2 tbsps of olive oil
- 3 pieces of garlic, crushed
- Zest of 1 lemon
- Juice of 1 lemon
- 1/4 teacup of chicken or vegetable broth
- Salt and pepper as required
- Fresh parsley, severed, for garnish
- Grated Parmesan cheese (optional)

Preparation Steps: Using a spiralizer, create zucchini noodles from the zucchinis. Put them away. Inside a big griddle, warm the olive oil at med-high temp. Include the crushed garlic and sauté for around a min till fragrant. Include the skinned and deveined shrimp to the griddle. Cook for 2-3 mins on all sides till they turn pink and opaque. Take out the shrimp from the griddle and put them away. Inside the same griddle, include the zucchini noodles. Sauté for 2-3 mins till they start to soften. Return the cooked shrimp to the griddle with the zucchini noodles. Include the lemon zest, lemon juice, and chicken or vegetable broth. Cook for an extra 2-3 mins, allowing the flavors to blend. Season with salt and pepper as required. Serve the Lemon Garlic Shrimp and Zucchini Noodles in containers, garnished with fresh parsley and grated Parmesan cheese if wanted.

Nutritional Info: Calories: 250 kcal, Protein: 20g, Carb: 8g, Fat: 15g

6. Spicy Cauliflower and Chickpea Curry

(Setup Time: 15 mins | Cooked in: 30 mins | How Many People: 4)

This curry provides a hearty and flavorful meal while adhering to the principles of a ketogenic diet. Cauliflower and chickpeas offer fiber and essential nutrients, while coconut milk provides healthy fats. The dish is rich in flavor and can be served over cauliflower rice for a low-carb option or enjoyed with naan bread for those who can afford a few extra carbs.

Recipe Components:

- 1 big cauliflower, cut into florets
- 1 can (15 oz.) of chickpeas, drained and washed
- 2 tbsps of vegetable oil
- 1 big onion, finely severed
- 2 pieces of garlic, crushed
- 1-inch piece of ginger, grated
- 1 can (14 oz.) of cubed tomatoes
- 2 tbsps of curry paste (adjust to your preferred level of spiciness)
- 1 can (14 oz.) of coconut milk
- Salt and pepper as required
- Fresh cilantro, severed, for garnish
- Cooked rice or naan bread for presenting

Preparation Steps: Inside a big griddle, warm the vegetable oil at med temp. Include the severed onion and cook for around 5 mins till it becomes translucent. Include the crushed garlic and grated ginger to the griddle. Sauté for an extra 2 mins till fragrant. Stir in the curry paste and cook for a min to release its flavors. Include the cauliflower florets and chickpeas to the griddle. Cook for 5 mins, mixing irregularly. Pour in the cubed tomatoes and coconut milk. Bring the mixture to a gentle simmer. Cover the griddle and let the curry simmer for around 15-20 mins, or till the cauliflower is soft. Season with salt and pepper as required. Serve the Spicy Cauliflower and Chickpea Curry over cooked rice or with naan bread. Garnish with fresh cilantro.

Nutritional Info: Calories: 350 kcal, Protein: 10g, Carb: 30g, Fat: 20g

7. Pesto and Prosciutto-Wrapped Asparagus
(Setup Time: 10 mins | Cooked in: 15 mins | How Many People: 4)

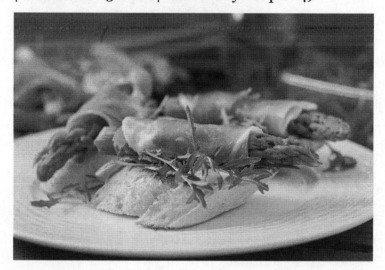

This recipe offers a delightful combination of flavors and textures, with asparagus providing fiber and essential nutrients, wrapped in prosciutto for added protein and flavor. With minimal carbs and ample healthy fats from olive oil and prosciutto, it's a perfect dish for seniors following a ketogenic lifestyle.

Recipe Components:

- 1 bunch of fresh asparagus spears
- 4 slices of prosciutto
- 4 tbsps of pesto sauce
- Olive oil for drizzling
- Salt and black pepper as required
- Grated Parmesan cheese (optional, for garnish)

Preparation Steps: Warm up your oven to 400 deg.F (200 deg.C). Wash and trim the tough ends of the asparagus spears. Lay out a slice of prosciutto on a clean surface. Spread a tbsp of pesto sauce over the prosciutto slice. Place several asparagus spears at the edge of the prosciutto slice and roll them up in the prosciutto. Repeat this process for the rest of the asparagus spears. Put the prosciutto-wrapped asparagus on a baking sheet. Spray a bit of olive oil over the asparagus bundles and season with salt and black pepper.

Bake in the warmed up oven for around 12-15 mins or till the asparagus is soft and the prosciutto is crispy. Garnish with grated Parmesan cheese if wanted.

Nutritional Info: Calories: 120 kcal, Protein: 6g, Carb: 3g, Fat: 10g

8. Lemon Butter Baked Cod with Herbed Tomatoes

(Setup Time: 10 mins | Cooked in: 20 mins | How Many People: 4)

Cod is a lean source of protein, and this dish incorporates healthy fats from butter and olive oil. Tomatoes offer antioxidants and flavor without adding excessive carbs. The dish is easy to prepare and bursting with freshness. It can be served with a side of steamed vegetables or cauliflower mash for a complete keto-friendly meal.

Recipe Components:

- 4 cod fillets
- 2 teacups cherry tomatoes, halved
- 4 tbsps unsalted butter, dissolved
- 2 pieces garlic, crushed
- Zest and juice of 1 lemon
- 2 tbsps fresh basil, severed
- 2 tbsps fresh parsley, severed
- Salt and black pepper as required
- Olive oil for drizzling

Preparation Steps: Warm up your oven to 375 deg.F (190 deg.C). Inside a baking dish, arrange the cod fillets and cherry tomato halves. Inside a small container, blend the dissolved butter, crushed garlic, lemon zest, and half of the lemon juice. Mix well. Spray the lemon butter mixture over the cod fillets and tomatoes. Spray the fresh basil and parsley over the top and season with salt and black pepper. Spray a bit of olive oil over the components. Bake in the warmed up oven for approximately 20 mins, or till the cod is fully cooked and the tomatoes are soft. Before presenting, spray the rest of the lemon juice over the dish for a fresh burst of flavor.

Nutritional Info: Calories: 240 kcal, Protein: 25g, Carb: 6g, Fat: 13g

9. Stuffed Zucchini Boats with Ground Turkey

(Setup Time: 15 mins | Cooked in: 35 mins | How Many People: 4)

This dish is versatile and can be customized with various herbs and spices. With zucchini as the base, this recipe provides essential nutrients and fiber while keeping carb intake low. It's a filling and nutritious option for seniors following a ketogenic diet.

Recipe Components:

- 4 medium zucchinis
- 1 lb. ground turkey
- 1 small onion, finely severed
- 2 pieces garlic, crushed
- 1 bell pepper, cubed
- 1 teacup cubed tomatoes
- 1 tsp dried oregano
- 1 tsp dried basil
- Salt and black pepper as required
- 1 teacup shredded mozzarella cheese
- Fresh parsley, for garnish

Preparation Steps: Warm up your oven to 375 deg.F (190 deg.C). Cut the zucchinis in half lengthwise and scoop out the centers to create "boats." Chop the scooped zucchini flesh and put it away. Inside a big griddle, heat some olive oil at med temp. Include the severed onion, garlic, and bell pepper. Sauté till they become soft. Include the ground turkey to the griddle and cook till it's browned and fully cooked. Include the cubed tomatoes, dried oregano, dried basil, salt, and black pepper to the griddle. Stir in the severed zucchini flesh. Cook for a couple of more mins till everything is thoroughly mixed. Fill each zucchini boat with the ground turkey mixture. Put the stuffed zucchini boats in a baking dish. Spray shredded mozzarella cheese over the top. Cover the baking dish with foil and bake for approximately 25 mins. Take out the foil and bake for an extra 10 mins or till the cheese is bubbly and golden. Garnish with fresh parsley and serve.

Nutritional Info: Calories: 280 kcal, Protein: 30g, Carb: 10g, Fat: 14g

10. Creamy Spinach and Artichoke Stuffed Chicken Breasts
(Setup Time: 20 mins | Cooked in: 25 mins | How Many People: 4)

This dish combines tender chicken breasts with a creamy spinach and artichoke filling, providing protein, healthy fats, and essential nutrients. The recipe is straightforward to prepare and can be served with a side of roasted vegetables or a green salad for a complete keto-friendly meal.

Recipe Components:

- 4 boneless, skinless chicken breasts
- 1 teacup fresh spinach, severed
- 1/2 teacup artichoke hearts, severed
- 1/2 teacup cream cheese
- 1/4 teacup grated Parmesan cheese
- 2 pieces garlic, crushed
- 1/2 tsp dried basil
- Salt and black pepper as required
- 2 tbsps olive oil
- 1 teacup chicken broth
- Fresh parsley, for garnish

Preparation Steps: Warm up your oven to 375 deg.F (190 deg.C). Inside a blending container, blend severed spinach, severed artichoke hearts, cream cheese, grated Parmesan cheese, crushed garlic, dried basil, salt, and black pepper. Mix till thoroughly mixed. Carefully slice a pocket into each chicken breast. Take cautions not to sever the whole thing with your knife. Stuff each chicken breast with the spinach and artichoke mixture. Inside an ovenproof griddle, warm olive oil at med-high temp. Include the stuffed chicken breasts and cook for around 3-4 mins on all sides till they're mildly browned. Pour the chicken broth into the griddle. Transfer the griddle to the warmed up oven and bake for around 15-20 mins or till the chicken is fully cooked and no longer pink in the center. Garnish with fresh parsley before presenting.

Nutritional Info: Calories: 350 kcal, Protein: 30g, Carb: 6g, Fat: 20

11. Roasted Garlic and Rosemary Lamb Chops

(Setup Time: 10 mins | Cooked in: 20 mins | How Many People: 4)

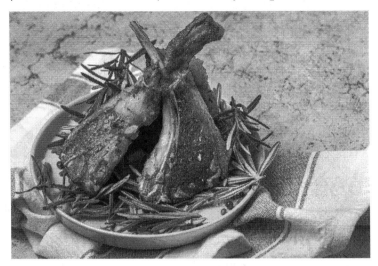

These lamb chops provide a rich source of protein and healthy fats, making them an ideal choice for seniors following a ketogenic diet. The garlic and rosemary add flavor without adding significant carbohydrates. This dish is easy to prepare and perfect for seniors looking for a flavorful and satisfying meal. It pairs well with a side of roasted vegetables or a simple salad for a complete keto-friendly dinner.

Recipe Components:

- 8 lamb chops
- 4 pieces of garlic, crushed
- 2 tbsps fresh rosemary, severed
- 2 tbsps olive oil
- Salt and black pepper as required
- 1 lemon, cut into wedges

Preparation Steps: Warm up your oven to 400 deg.F (200 deg.C). Inside a small container, blend the crushed garlic, severed rosemary, olive oil, salt, and black pepper. Rub the garlic and rosemary mixture evenly on both sides of the lamb chops. Heat an ovenproof griddle at med-high temp. Once hot, include the lamb chops and sear for around 2-3 mins on all sides till they're nicely browned. Transfer the griddle with the lamb chops to the warmed up oven. Roast for around 10-15 mins for medium-rare, or adjust the cooking time according to your desired level of doneness. Take out the lamb chops from the oven and let them rest for a couple of mins before presenting. Serve with lemon wedges on the side for an extra burst of flavor.

Nutritional Info: Calories: 300 kcal, Protein: 25g, Carb: 2g, Fat: 21g

12. Thai-inspired Coconut Shrimp Soup

(Setup Time: 10 mins | Cooked in: 20 mins | How Many People: 4)

This soup offers a flavorful blend of shrimp, coconut milk, and aromatic Thai spices. It provides a good source of protein and healthy fats, with minimal carbs, making it suitable for seniors on a ketogenic diet. The soup is quick and easy to prepare, making it a convenient option for busy seniors.

Recipe Components:

- 1 lb. big shrimp, skinned and deveined
- 1 can (14 oz.) coconut milk
- 3 teacups chicken broth
- 2 stalks lemongrass, cut into 2-inch pieces and smashed
- 3-4 slices galangal or ginger
- 2-3 kaffir lime leaves
- 1-2 red chili peppers, carved (adjust to your spice preference)
- 2-3 pieces garlic, crushed
- 1 small onion, carved
- 1 teacup mushrooms, carved
- 1-2 tbsps fish sauce (adjust as required)
- 1-2 tbsps lime juice (adjust as required)
- Fresh cilantro leaves for garnish
- Salt and sugar as required

Preparation Steps: Inside a big pot, heat the coconut milk and chicken broth at med temp. Include lemongrass, galangal or ginger, kaffir lime leaves, and bring to a gentle simmer. Let it simmer for around 5-10 mins to infuse the flavors. Include the carved onion, garlic, mushrooms, and red chili peppers to the pot. Cook for around 5 mins till the vegetables are soft. Stir in the shrimp and let them cook for 2-3 mins till they turn pink and opaque. Season the soup with fish sauce, lime juice, salt, and sugar as required. Adjust the seasoning as needed. Take out the lemongrass, galangal or ginger, and kaffir lime leaves from the soup. Ladle the hot soup into presenting containers. Garnish with fresh cilantro leaves.

Nutritional Info: Calories: 250-300 kcal, Protein: 20-25g, Carb: 5-10g, Fat: 15-20g

13. Keto Spaghetti Squash Carbonara

(Setup Time: 15 mins | Cooked in: 45 mins | How Many People: 4)

This dish offers all the flavors of traditional carbonara without the carbs. Spaghetti squash replaces pasta, providing a low-carb alternative, while bacon, eggs, and Parmesan cheese contribute protein and healthy fats. Seniors following a ketogenic diet can enjoy this comforting and satisfying dish without worrying about carb intake. It's a delicious option for dinner and can be customized with additional herbs and spices to suit individual tastes.

Recipe Components:

- 1 medium-sized spaghetti squash
- 4 slices of bacon, severed
- 2 pieces garlic, crushed
- 2 big eggs
- 1/2 teacup grated Parmesan cheese
- 1/4 teacup heavy cream
- Salt and black pepper as required
- Fresh parsley for garnish (optional)

Preparation Steps: Warm up your oven to 375 deg.F (190 deg.C). Cut the spaghetti squash in half lengthwise. Scoop out the seeds and place the halves, cut side down, on a baking sheet. Roast them in the oven for around 30-40 mins or till the flesh is soft. While the squash is roasting, cook the severed bacon in a griddle at med temp. till it's crispy.

Take out the bacon and put it away, leaving the bacon fat in the griddle. Inside the same griddle, include crushed garlic and sauté for a min till fragrant. Inside a container, whisk collectively the eggs, grated Parmesan cheese, and heavy cream. When the spaghetti squash is done, use a fork to scrape the flesh into "spaghetti" strands. Include the strands to the griddle with the garlic and bacon fat. Pour the egg and cheese mixture over the spaghetti squash, stirring quickly to blend. The heat of the squash will cook the eggs and create a creamy sauce. Season with salt and black pepper as required. Garnish with crispy bacon and fresh parsley, if wanted.

Nutritional Info: Calories: 350-400 kcal, Protein: 15-20g, Carb: 10-15g, Fat: 25-30g

14. Baked Dijon Mustard and Herb-Crusted Tilapia
(Setup Time: 10 mins | Cooked in: 15 mins | How Many People: 4)

Tilapia is a lean source of protein, and this dish is coated in a flavorful mixture of Dijon mustard, herbs, and almond meal. It provides a satisfying meal with minimal carbs, making it suitable for seniors following a ketogenic diet.

Recipe Components:

- 4 tilapia fillets
- 2 tbsps Dijon mustard
- 1/2 teacup almond meal (or almond flour)
- 2 tbsps fresh herbs (e.g., parsley, thyme, or rosemary), finely severed
- 2 pieces garlic, crushed
- 1/4 teacup grated Parmesan cheese
- Salt and black pepper as required
- Lemon wedges for presenting

Preparation Steps: Warm up your oven to 375 deg.F (190 deg.C). Inside a shallow container, blend collectively the almond meal, fresh herbs, crushed garlic, grated Parmesan cheese, salt, and black pepper. Brush each tilapia fillet with a layer of Dijon mustard. Press each fillet into the almond meal and herb mixture, covering it evenly on both sides. Put the covered fillets on a baking sheet lined with parchment paper. Bake in the warmed up oven for around 15 mins or till the fish flakes simply with a fork and the crust is golden brown. Serve the Dijon Mustard and Herb-Crusted Tilapia with lemon wedges for a zesty kick.

Nutritional Info: Calories: 200-250 kcal, Protein: 25-30g, Carb: 5-10g, Fat: 10-15g

15. Cabbage and Sausage Stir-Fry
(Setup Time: 10 mins | Cooked in: 20 mins | How Many People: 4)

This stir-fry combines cabbage and sausage for a hearty and flavorful dish. It's high in protein and healthy fats, with moderate carbs from the cabbage, making it suitable for seniors following a ketogenic diet. The stir-fry is quick and easy to prepare, making it a convenient option for busy seniors. It can be customized with additional vegetables or spices to suit individual preferences, providing a satisfying and nutritious meal option.

Recipe Components:

- 1 medium head of cabbage, finely cut
- 1 lb. sausage links, carved into rounds
- 1 onion, finely cut
- 2 pieces garlic, crushed
- 2 tbsps olive oil
- 1 tsp paprika
- Salt and black pepper as required
- Fresh parsley for garnish (optional)

Preparation Steps: Inside a big griddle or wok, warm the olive oil at med-high temp. Include the carved sausage rounds and cook till they start to brown, around 5 mins. Include the crushed garlic and carved onion, and sauté for an extra 3-4 mins till the onion becomes translucent. Spray the paprika over the sausage and vegetables, and stir well. Include the finely cut cabbage to the griddle and shake everything together. Cook for around 10-12 mins, or till the cabbage is soft and mildly caramelized. Season the stir-fry with salt and black pepper as required. Garnish with fresh parsley, if wanted.

Nutritional Info: Calories: 300-350 kcal, Protein: 15-20g, Carb: 10-15g, Fat: 20-25g

16. Keto Pork Chops with Blue Cheese Sauce

(Setup Time: 10 mins | Cooked in: 20 mins | How Many People: 4)

This dish offers protein-rich pork chops paired with a flavorful blue cheese sauce. With minimal carbs and plenty of healthy fats, it's an excellent choice for seniors following a ketogenic diet.

Recipe Components:

- 4 boneless pork chops
- Salt and black pepper as required
- 2 tbsps olive oil
- 1/2 teacup heavy cream
- 1/2 teacup blue cheese, crumbled
- 2 pieces garlic, crushed
- 1/2 teacup chicken broth
- 1 tbsp fresh parsley, severed, for garnish

Preparation Steps: Season the pork chops with salt and black pepper on both sides. Inside a big griddle, warm the olive oil at med-high temp. Include the pork chops and cook for around 4-5 mins on all sides, or till they are fully cooked and golden brown. Take out the pork chops from the griddle and put them away. Inside the same griddle, include the crushed garlic and sauté for around 1 min. Pour in the chicken broth and bring it to a simmer. Scrape up any browned bits from the bottom of the pan. Reduce the heat and stir in the heavy cream. Let it simmer for a couple of mins till it densess mildly. Include the crumbled blue cheese and stir till it dissolves into the sauce. Return the pork chops to the griddle and let them heat through in the sauce for a couple of mins. Garnish with severed fresh parsley before presenting.

Nutritional Info: Calories: 400-450 kcal, Protein: 30-35g, Carb: 2-4g, Fat: 30-35g

17. Keto Pesto and Mozzarella Stuffed Chicken

(Setup Time: 15 mins | Cooked in: 25 mins | How Many People: 4)

These stuffed chicken breasts are filled with keto-friendly pesto and mozzarella cheese, providing a satisfying meal with minimal carbs. High in protein and healthy fats, they're ideal for seniors following a ketogenic diet. This dish is simple to prepare and can be customized with additional herbs and spices to suit individual tastes. Baking the chicken breasts ensures they're cooked through while keeping them tender and juicy.

Recipe Components:

- 4 boneless, skinless chicken breasts
- Salt and black pepper as required
- 1/2 teacup keto-friendly pesto sauce
- 1 teacup mozzarella cheese, shredded
- 2 tbsps olive oil
- 1 tsp Italian seasoning (optional)
- Fresh basil leaves for garnish (optional)

Preparation Steps: Warm up your oven to 375 deg.F (190 deg.C). Place the chicken breasts on a clean surface and lay them out flat. Using a sharp knife, carefully cut a pocket into every chicken breast in a horizontal direction, taking care not to cut through to the opposite side. Season the inside of each chicken breast with salt and black pepper. Stuff each chicken breast with 2 tbsps of keto-friendly pesto sauce and 1/4 teacup of mozzarella cheese. Close the pockets by securing them with toothpicks to keep the filling in. Season the outside of each chicken breast with salt, black pepper, and Italian seasoning if wanted. Inside an ovenproof griddle, warm the olive oil at med-high temp. Include the stuffed chicken breasts and cook for around 3-4 mins on all sides or till they are golden brown. Transfer the griddle to the warmed up oven and bake for around 15-20 mins or till the chicken is fully cooked and the cheese is dissolved and bubbly. Garnish with fresh basil leaves if wanted and serve.

Nutritional Info: Calories: 350-400 kcal, Protein: 30-35g, Carb: 2-4g, Fat: 20-25g

18. Lemon Herb Shrimp and Zucchini Noodles

(Setup Time: 15 mins | Cooked in: 10 mins | How Many People: 4)

This dish features shrimp and zucchini noodles in a flavorful lemon herb sauce. Low in carbs and high in protein, it's a nutritious and satisfying option for seniors following a ketogenic diet. Quick to prepare and bursting with fresh flavors, this dish is perfect for busy seniors. The zucchini noodles add bulk without adding significant carbs, making it a light and refreshing meal option.

Recipe Components:

- 1 lb. big shrimp, skinned and deveined
- 4 medium zucchinis
- 2 tbsps olive oil
- 3 pieces garlic, crushed
- Zest and juice of 1 lemon
- 2 tbsps fresh basil, severed

- 2 tbsps fresh parsley, severed
- Salt and black pepper as required
- Grated Parmesan cheese for garnish (optional)

Preparation Steps: Using a spiralizer, create zucchini noodles from the zucchinis. Put them away. Inside a big griddle, warm the olive oil at med-high temp. Include the crushed garlic and sauté for around 1 min till fragrant. Include the shrimp to the griddle and cook for 2-3 mins on all sides till they turn pink and opaque. Season with salt and black pepper. Take out the cooked shrimp from the griddle and put them away. Inside the same griddle, include the zucchini noodles and cook for around 2-3 mins till they are fully heated and mildly soft. Return the cooked shrimp to the griddle. Include the lemon zest, lemon juice, fresh basil, and fresh parsley. Shake everything together to blend. Season with additional salt and black pepper if needed. Serve hot, garnished with grated Parmesan cheese if wanted.

Nutritional Info: Calories: 200-250 kcal, Protein: 20-25g, Carb: 10-12g, Fat: 8-10g

19. Beef and Broccoli Stir-Fry with Sesame Seeds
(Setup Time: 15 mins | Cooked in: 15 mins | How Many People: 4)

This stir-fry combines tender beef, crisp broccoli, and a flavorful sauce, offering a satisfying meal with minimal carbs. High in protein and healthy fats, it's a nutritious option for seniors following a ketogenic diet. Easy to make and full of flavor, this stir-fry is perfect for seniors looking for a quick and convenient meal option. Serve it over cauliflower rice for a complete keto-friendly meal.

Recipe Components:

- 1 lb. flank steak, finely cut
- 2 teacups broccoli florets
- 2 tbsps sesame oil
- 3 pieces garlic, crushed
- 1 tbsp ginger, crushed
- 1/4 teacup low-sodium soy sauce
- 2 tbsps oyster sauce
- 1 tbsp brown sugar or a sugar substitute for a keto-friendly option
- 2 tbsps sesame seeds
- Salt and black pepper as required
- Red pepper flakes for a spicy kick (optional)
- Sliced green onions for garnish (optional)

Preparation Steps: Inside a container, blend the soy sauce, oyster sauce, brown sugar (or substitute), and put it away. Heat 1 tbsp of sesame oil in a big griddle or wok at med-high temp. Include the carved flank steak and stir-fry for 2-3 mins till it's browned. Take out the beef from the griddle and put it away. Inside the same griddle, include the rest of the sesame oil and heat it. Include the crushed garlic and ginger, and sauté for around 30 secs till fragrant. Include the broccoli florets to the griddle and stir-fry for 3-4 mins till they are soft-crisp. Return the cooked beef to the griddle and pour the sauce over it. Stir everything together and cook for an extra 2-3 mins till the sauce denses and covers the beef and broccoli. Season with salt, black pepper, and red pepper flakes if wanted. Spray sesame seeds on top and garnish with carved green onions. Serve hot over cauliflower rice or enjoy it on its own.

Nutritional Info: Calories: 300-350 kcal, Protein: 25-30g, Carb: 10-12g, Fat: 15-20g

20. Stuffed Avocado with Tuna and Olive Tapenade

(Setup Time: 10 mins | How Many People: 2)

These stuffed avocados are filled with a flavorful mixture of tuna and olive tapenade, providing a satisfying meal with minimal carbs. High in healthy fats and protein, they're an excellent option for seniors following a ketogenic diet.

Recipe Components:

- 2 ripe avocados
- 1 can (5 oz) of tuna, drained
- 2 tbsps of olive tapenade
- 1 tbsp of lemon juice
- 2 tbsps of severed fresh parsley
- Salt and black pepper as required
- Red pepper flakes for a bit of heat (optional)
- Lemon wedges for garnish (optional)

Preparation Steps:

✓ Cut the avocados in half and take out the pits. Scoop out a small portion of the flesh from each avocado half to create a hollow space for the filling.

✓ Inside a blending container, blend the drained tuna, olive tapenade, lemon juice, and severed fresh parsley. Mix well to create the filling.

✓ Season the filling with a tweak of salt and black pepper. Include red pepper flakes if you prefer a bit of heat.

✓ Stuff each avocado half with the tuna and olive tapenade filling, dividing it equally between the halves.

✓ Garnish with lemon wedges and additional severed parsley if wanted.

✓ Serve instantly as a delicious and healthy keto-friendly appetizer or light meal.

Nutritional Info: Calories: 250-300 kcal, Protein: 15-20g, Carb: 10-12g, Fat: 15-20g

Chapter 9: Keto Recipes For Dessert & Snacks

1. Coconut Almond Butter Bites
(Setup Time: 15 mins | 12 bites)

These bites are low in carbs and high in healthy fats, making them suitable for a ketogenic diet. They provide a quick energy boost without causing spikes in blood sugar levels. Simple to prepare and requiring minimal ingredients, these coconut almond butter bites are an easy snack option for seniors. They can be made ahead of time and stored in the fridge for a convenient grab-and-go snack.

Recipe Components:

- 1/2 teacup almond butter
- 1/4 teacup unsweetened shredded coconut
- 1/4 teacup almond flour
- 2 tbsps coconut oil, dissolved
- 2 tbsps keto-friendly sweetener (e.g., erythritol or stevia)
- 1/2 tsp vanilla extract
- A tweak of salt

Preparation Steps: Inside a blending container, blend almond butter, unsweetened shredded coconut, almond flour, dissolved coconut oil, keto-friendly sweetener, vanilla extract, and a tweak of salt. Mix the entire components till they form a dough-like consistency. Using your hands, roll the mixture into small bite-sized balls. Put the bites on a parchment paper-lined tray or plate. Chill in the fridge for almost 30 mins to firm up. Once the bites have set, they are ready to enjoy.

Nutritional Info: Calories: 97, Fat: 8g, Protein: 3g, Carb: 3g, Fiber: 2g, Net Carbs: 1g

2. Pumpkin Spice Keto Cookies
(Setup Time: 15 mins | Cooked in: 12-15 mins | 12 cookies)

These cookies are keto-friendly and low in carbs, making them suitable for seniors following a ketogenic diet. The pumpkin spice adds flavor without adding unnecessary sugars.

Recipe Components:

- 1 teacup almond flour
- 1/4 teacup canned pumpkin
- 1/4 teacup keto-friendly sweetener (e.g., erythritol or stevia)
- 1/4 teacup dissolved coconut oil
- 1 tsp pumpkin pie spice
- 1/2 tsp vanilla extract
- 1/4 tsp baking powder
- A tweak of salt

Preparation Steps: Warm up your oven to 350 deg.F (175 deg.C) and line a baking sheet with parchment paper. Inside a blending container, blend almond flour, canned pumpkin, keto-friendly sweetener, dissolved coconut oil, pumpkin pie spice, vanilla extract, baking powder, and a tweak of salt. Mix till a dough forms.

Using your hands, form the dough into 12 small cookie shapes and put them on the prepared baking sheet. Gently flatten each cookie with a fork. Bake in the warmed up oven for 12-15 mins or till the cookies are mildly golden around the edges. Take out from the oven and let the cookies cool on the baking sheet for a couple of mins, then transfer them to a wire stand to cool entirely.

Nutritional Info: Calories: 90, Fat: 8g, Protein: 2g, Carb: 3g, Fiber: 1g, Net Carbs: 2g

3. Matcha Green Tea Fat Bombs

(Setup Time: 10 mins | Cooked in: 1h | 12 fat bombs)

These fat bombs are high in healthy fats and low in carbs, making them an ideal snack for seniors on a ketogenic diet. The matcha green tea powder provides antioxidants and flavor without adding extra carbs. Quick and easy to make, these matcha green tea fat bombs can be prepared ahead of time and stored in the freezer for a convenient snack option. They're perfect for satisfying hunger between meals or as a pre-workout energy boost.

Recipe Components:

- 1/2 teacup coconut oil
- 1/4 teacup unsweetened almond butter
- 2 tbsps matcha green tea powder
- 2 tbsps powdered Erythritol (or your preferred keto-friendly sweetener)
- 1/2 tsp vanilla extract
- A tweak of salt

Preparation Steps: Inside a microwave-safe container, dissolve the coconut oil and almond butter together. You can do this by microwaving in 20-second intervals till fully dissolved or using a double boiler. Once dissolved, stir in the matcha green tea powder, powdered Erythritol, vanilla extract, and a tweak of salt. Mix till the mixture is smooth and thoroughly mixed. Using a silicone mold or an ice cube tray, pour the mixture into individual mold sections. You can also use silicone molds for fun shapes. Put the mold in the freezer for almost 1 hr or till the fat bombs are firm. Once set, take out the fat bombs from the mold and store them in a sealed container in the freezer.

Nutritional Info: Calories: 90, Fat: 9g, Protein: 1g, Carb: 1g, Fiber: 1g, Net Carbs: 0g

4. Keto Peanut Butter Fudge

(Setup Time: 10 mins | Chilling: 2h | 16 pieces)

This peanut butter fudge is keto-friendly and low in carbs, making it suitable for seniors following a ketogenic diet. It provides a sweet treat without spiking blood sugar levels. It can be made ahead of time and stored in the fridge for a quick and easy treat.

Recipe Components:

- 1 teacup natural peanut butter (unsweetened)
- 1/2 teacup coconut oil
- 1/4 teacup powdered Erythritol (or your preferred keto-friendly sweetener)
- 1/2 tsp vanilla extract

- A tweak of salt

Preparation Steps: Inside a microwave-safe container, dissolve the coconut oil and natural peanut butter together. You can do this by microwaving in 20-second intervals till fully dissolved or using a double boiler. Once dissolved, stir in the powdered Erythritol, vanilla extract, and a tweak of salt. Mix till the mixture is smooth and thoroughly mixed. Line a small square or rectangular dish with parchment paper, leaving some excess paper hanging over the sides for easy removal. Pour the peanut butter mixture into the dish and disperse it out uniformly. Put the dish in the fridge for around 2 hrs, or till the fudge is firm. Once set, use the parchment paper to lift the fudge out of the dish. Cut it into 16 equal pieces. Store the keto peanut butter fudge in the fridge.

Nutritional Info: Calories: 140, Fat: 12g, Protein: 4g, Carb: 3g, Fiber: 2g, Net Carbs: 1g

5. Blueberry Almond Keto Granola

(Setup Time: 10 mins | Cooked in: 25 mins | How Many People: 8)

This granola is low in carbs and high in healthy fats, making it suitable for a ketogenic diet. The addition of blueberries provides antioxidants and flavor without adding extra carbs. It can be enjoyed with yogurt or milk or eaten on its own for a crunchy and satisfying snack.

Recipe Components:

- 1 teacup almond slices
- 1/2 teacup unsweetened shredded coconut
- 1/2 teacup chia seeds
- 1/4 teacup flaxseeds
- 1/4 teacup sunflower seeds
- 1/4 teacup pumpkin seeds
- 1/4 teacup erythritol (or your preferred keto-friendly sweetener)
- 1/4 teacup coconut oil, dissolved
- 1 tsp vanilla extract
- 1/2 teacup freeze-dried blueberries

Preparation Steps: Warm up your oven to 325 deg.F (160 deg.C) and line a baking sheet with parchment paper. Inside a big blending container, blend almond slices, unsweetened shredded coconut, chia seeds, flaxseeds, sunflower seeds, pumpkin seeds, and erythritol. Inside a separate microwave-safe container, dissolve the coconut oil. Stir in the vanilla extract. Pour the dissolved coconut oil mixture over the dry components in the big mixing container. Mix well till everything is evenly covered. Spread the granola mixture evenly on the prepared baking sheet. Bake in the warmed up oven for around 20-25 mins, or till it turns golden brown, stirring once or twice during baking for even browning. Take out from the oven and let the granola cool entirely on the baking sheet. Once the granola has cooled, break it into clusters and mix in the freeze-dried blueberries. Store the Blueberry Almond Keto Granola in a sealed container.

Nutritional Info: Calories: 272, Fat: 23g, Protein: 6g, Carb: 11g, Fiber: 6g, Net Carbs: 5g

6. Chocolate Mint Avocado Pudding

(Setup Time: 10 mins | How Many People: 4)

Quick to prepare and requiring minimal ingredients, this pudding is easy on the digestive system and can be enjoyed by seniors with varying dietary needs.

Avocado provides healthy fats and fiber, while cocoa powder adds antioxidants. The addition of mint extract adds a refreshing twist to the dessert.

Recipe Components:

- 2 ripe avocados
- 1/4 teacup unsweetened cocoa powder
- 1/4 teacup almond milk (or any keto-friendly milk of your choice)
- 1/4 teacup keto-friendly sweetener (e.g., erythritol or stevia)
- 1/2 tsp mint extract
- A tweak of salt
- Whipped cream and fresh mint leaves for garnish (optional)

Preparation Steps: Cut the avocados in half, take out the pits, and scoop out the flesh into a blender or food processor. Include the unsweetened cocoa powder, almond milk, keto-friendly sweetener, mint extract, and a tweak of salt to the blender. Blend the entire components till you achieve a smooth and creamy consistency. You may need to scrape down the sides and blend again to ensure everything is well mixed. Taste the pudding and adjust the sweetness or mint flavor to your liking. Once the pudding is smooth and the taste is to your preference, transfer it to presenting dishes or teacups. Put in the fridge for almost 30 mins to chill and set. Serve chilled, optionally garnished with a dollop of whipped cream and a fresh mint leaf.

Nutritional Info: Calories: 174, Fat: 15g, Protein: 2g, Carb: 10g, Fiber: 7g, Net Carbs: 3g

7. Cinnamon Pecan Keto Brittle

(Setup Time: 10 mins | Cooked in: 20 mins | How Many People: 8)

This brittle offers a crunchy texture with a sweet cinnamon flavor, making it a delightful snack for seniors on a ketogenic diet. Pecans provide healthy fats and protein, while cinnamon adds warmth and depth of flavor. Simple to make and perfect for satisfying cravings for something crunchy and sweet, this keto brittle is a great alternative to traditional sugary snacks. It can be made in batches and stored for easy snacking.

Recipe Components:

- 1 teacup pecan halves
- 1/4 teacup unsalted butter
- 1/4 teacup keto-friendly sweetener (e.g., erythritol or stevia)
- 1 tsp ground cinnamon
- 1/4 tsp vanilla extract
- A tweak of salt

Preparation Steps: Warm up your oven to 325 deg.F (163 deg.C) and line a baking sheet with parchment paper. Inside a griddle at med temp., dissolve the unsalted butter. Stir in the keto-friendly sweetener, ground cinnamon, and a tweak of salt. Continue to cook and stir till the sweetener has entirely dissolved and the mixture is thoroughly mixed. Take out the griddle from heat and stir in the vanilla extract. Include the pecan halves to the griddle and cover them evenly with the cinnamon mixture. Spread the covered pecans onto the prepared baking sheet in a single layer. Bake in the warmed up oven for around 20 mins, or till the pecans are toasted and the syrup has densesed. Take out from the oven and let it cool entirely. As it cools, the mixture will harden and form a brittle. Once fully cooled and set, break the brittle into pieces. Store in a sealed container.

Nutritional Info: Calories: 175, Fat: 18g, Protein: 1g, Carb: 2g, Fiber: 1g, Net Carbs: 1g

8. Vanilla Chia Pudding with Berries
(Setup Time: 5 mins (plus chilling time) | How Many People: 2)

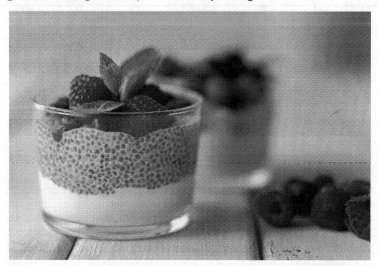

This pudding offers a creamy texture with a hint of vanilla sweetness, making it a versatile dessert or breakfast option for seniors on a ketogenic diet. Chia seeds provide fiber and omega-3 fatty acids, while berries add antioxidants and natural sweetness. Easy to prepare and customizable with different types of berries, this chia pudding is a nutritious and delicious option for seniors looking to increase their intake of healthy fats and fiber.

Recipe Components:

- 1/4 teacup chia seeds
- 1 teacup unsweetened almond milk (or any preferred milk)
- 1/2 tsp pure vanilla extract
- 1 tbsp keto-friendly sweetener (e.g., erythritol or stevia), or as required
- 1/2 teacup mixed berries (strawberries, blueberries, raspberries)
- Fresh mint leaves for garnish (optional)

Preparation Steps: Inside a blending container, blend the chia seeds, unsweetened almond milk, pure vanilla extract, and the keto-friendly sweetener. Mix well to ensure there are no clumps. Let the mixture sit for a couple of mins and then stir it again to prevent clumping. You can adjust the sweetness to your preference by adding more sweetener if needed. Cover the container and put in the fridge the chia pudding mixture for almost 2 hrs or overnight. It's ready when the chia seeds have absorbed the liquid and the mixture has densesed. When you're ready to serve, give the pudding a good stir. If it has densesed too much, you can include a little more almond milk to achieve your anticipated uniformity. Split the chia pudding into two presenting glasses. Top each presenting with the mixed berries and garnish with fresh mint leaves if wanted. Enjoy your Vanilla Chia Pudding with Berries as a delightful keto-friendly dessert or breakfast.

Nutritional Info: Calories: 150, Fat: 8g, Protein: 4g, Carb: 14g, Fiber: 10g, Net Carbs: 4g

9. Keto Cheesecake Bites

(Setup Time: 15 mins (plus chilling time) | 12 bites)

These cheesecake bites offer a rich and creamy texture with a sweet vanilla flavor, making them a decadent dessert option for seniors on a ketogenic diet. Cream cheese provides healthy fats and protein, while almond flour adds texture and flavor. Although they require chilling time, these cheesecake bites are relatively easy to make and can be prepared ahead of time for special occasions or gatherings. They can be customized with different toppings or flavors to suit individual preferences.

Recipe Components:

For the Crust:

- 1/2 teacup almond flour
- 2 tbsps unsweetened cocoa powder
- 2 tbsps keto-friendly sweetener (e.g., erythritol or stevia)
- 2 tbsps dissolved unsalted butter

For the Cheesecake Filling:

- 8 oz. cream cheese, softened
- 1/4 teacup keto-friendly sweetener
- 1 tsp pure vanilla extract
- 1/4 teacup heavy cream

For Topping:

- Sugar-free chocolate chips (optional)

Preparation Steps:

For the Crust: Inside a blending container, blend almond flour, unsweetened cocoa powder, keto-friendly sweetener, and dissolved unsalted butter. Mix till it forms a crumbly mixture. Line a muffin tin with cupcake liners. Split the crust mixture evenly among the cupcake liners, pressing it down to form the crust for each cheesecake bite.

For the Cheesecake Filling: Inside a distinct container, beat the softened cream cheese, keto-friendly sweetener, and pure vanilla extract till smooth and creamy. Include the heavy cream and mix till thoroughly mixed. Spoon the cheesecake filling over the crust in each cupcake liner, filling them almost to the top.

Chilling: If desired, spray a couple of sugar-free chocolate chips on top of each cheesecake bite. Put the muffin tin in the fridge and let the cheesecake bites chill for almost 2 hrs, or till they are set. Once set, take out them from the muffin tin and serve. Enjoy your keto cheesecake bites!

Nutritional Info: Calories: 138, Fat: 13g, Protein: 2g, Carb: 3g, Fiber: 1g, Net Carbs: 2g

10. Peanut Butter Chocolate Chip Keto Bars

(Setup Time: 10 mins | Cooked in: 20 mins | 12 bars)

These bars offer a chewy texture with a combination of peanut butter and chocolate flavors, making them a satisfying snack for seniors on a ketogenic diet. Peanut butter provides protein and healthy fats, while almond flour adds texture and fiber. They can be stored in the fridge or freezer for longer shelf life.

Recipe Components:

- 1 teacup natural peanut butter (no added sugar)
- 1/4 teacup keto-friendly sweetener (e.g., erythritol or stevia)
- 1 big egg
- 1 tsp pure vanilla extract
- 1/2 teacup almond flour
- 1/4 teacup unsweetened cocoa powder
- 1/2 tsp baking powder
- 1/4 teacup sugar-free chocolate chips

Preparation Steps: Warm up your oven to 350 deg.F (175 deg.C) and line an 8x8-inch (20x20 cm) baking pan with parchment paper. Inside a blending container, blend the natural peanut butter, keto-friendly sweetener, egg, and pure vanilla extract. Mix till the entire components are well incorporated. Inside a distinct container, whisk collectively the almond flour, unsweetened cocoa powder, and baking powder. Slowly include the dry components to the peanut butter mixture and mix till a dense batter forms. Wrap in the sugar-free chocolate chips. Transfer the batter to the prepared baking pan and disperse it out uniformly. Bake in the warmed up oven for around 20 mins or till the edges are set, and a toothpick immersed into the middle comes out with just a couple of moist crumbs. Take out from the oven and allow the bars to cool in the pan for around 10 mins. Lift the bars out of the pan using the parchment paper and let them cool entirely on a wire stand. Once cool, cut into 12 bars and enjoy your Peanut Butter Chocolate Chip Keto Bars!

Nutritional Info: Calories: 170, Fat: 13g, Protein: 6g, Carb: 7g, Fiber: 3g, Net Carbs: 4g

11. Salted Caramel Fat Bombs

(Setup Time: 10 mins | 12 fat bombs)

These fat bombs offer a rich and creamy caramel flavor with a hint of saltiness, making them a satisfying keto-friendly treat for seniors. They are easy to make and can be stored in the freezer for quick snacking.

Recipe Components:

- 1/2 teacup unsalted butter, softened
- 1/4 teacup coconut oil

- 1/4 teacup sugar-free caramel syrup
- 1 tsp vanilla extract
- 1/4 tsp sea salt
- 1/4 teacup almond butter
- 1/4 teacup powdered erythritol (or your preferred keto-friendly sweetener)

Preparation Steps: Inside a blending container, blend the softened unsalted butter, coconut oil, sugar-free caramel syrup, vanilla extract, and sea salt. Mix till the entire components are thoroughly mixed. Include the almond butter and powdered erythritol to the mixture. Stir till you have a smooth and creamy caramel-like mixture. Line a mini-muffin tin or a silicone mold with 12 cavities. Spoon the caramel mixture into each cavity, filling them around 2/3 full. Put the mold in the freezer and allow the fat bombs to set for almost 2 hrs. Once they are firm, take out the fat bombs from the mold and store them in a sealed container in the freezer. Enjoy your Salted Caramel Fat Bombs straight from the freezer as a delightful keto-friendly treat!

Nutritional Info: Calories: 118, Fat: 12g, Protein: 0.5g, Carb: 1g, Fiber: 0.5g, Net Carbs: 0.5g

12. Chocolate Dipped Macadamia Nut Bites

(Setup Time: 15 mins | Cooked in: 0 mins (no baking required) | 12 macadamia nut bites)

Quick and easy to make without requiring any baking, these macadamia nut bites are suitable for seniors who prefer simple recipes with minimal preparation time. Macadamia nuts are high in healthy fats, while dark chocolate adds antioxidants. They can be customized with optional toppings for added flavor and texture.

Recipe Components:

- 1 teacup roasted macadamia nuts
- 1/4 teacup sugar-free dark chocolate chips
- 1 tbsp coconut oil
- 1/2 tsp vanilla extract
- A tweak of sea salt (optional)

Preparation Steps: Inside a microwave-safe container, blend the sugar-free dark chocolate chips and coconut oil. Microwave in 20-second intervals, stirring between each interval, till the chocolate is fully dissolved and smooth. Stir in the vanilla extract and a tweak of sea salt, if wanted, into the dissolved chocolate mixture. Put a sheet of parchment paper on a baking sheet or tray. Dip each roasted macadamia nut into the chocolate mixture, ensuring it's covered evenly, and place it on the parchment paper. Once the entire macadamia nuts are covered, put the baking sheet in the fridge for around 20-30 mins, or till the chocolate hardens. Once the chocolate is set, take out the macadamia nut bites from the parchment paper, and they're ready to enjoy. Store any leftovers in a sealed container in the fridge.

Nutritional Info: Calories: 95, Fat: 9.5g, Protein: 1g, Carb: 2g, Fiber: 1.5g, Net Carbs: 0.5g

13. Coconut Lime Energy Bites

(Setup Time: 15 mins | Cooked in: 0 mins (no baking required) | 12 energy bites)

These energy bites offer a refreshing combination of coconut and lime flavors, providing a burst of energy without the need for refined sugars.

The addition of chia seeds adds fiber and omega-3 fatty acids. They can be stored in the fridge for easy access and enjoyed throughout the day.

Recipe Components:

- 1 teacup unsweetened shredded coconut
- 1/2 teacup almond flour
- Zest and juice of 1 lime
- 2 tbsps coconut oil (dissolved)
- 2 tbsps Erythritol or your preferred keto-friendly sweetener
- 1 tsp vanilla extract
- A tweak of salt

Preparation Steps: Inside a blending container, blend the unsweetened shredded coconut and almond flour. Include the lime zest and lime juice to the dry components, followed by the dissolved coconut oil, Erythritol (or sweetener of your choice), vanilla extract, and a tweak of salt. Mix the components till thoroughly mixed. The mixture should be mildly sticky and simply moldable. Take small portions of the mixture and roll them into bite-sized balls, about 1 inch in diameter. Put the energy bites on a plate or tray lined with parchment paper. Let the energy bites set in the fridge for almost 30 mins to firm up. Once they've hardened, transfer them to a sealed container for storage.

Nutritional Info: Calories: 76, Fat: 7g, Protein: 1g, Carb: 3g, Fiber: 2g, Net Carbs: 1g

14. Keto Tiramisu Fat Bombs
(Setup Time: 20 mins | Cooked in: 0 mins (no baking required) | 12 fat bombs)

These fat bombs offer the flavors of traditional tiramisu in a keto-friendly format, making them a decadent treat for seniors on a ketogenic diet. Mascarpone cheese provides richness, while espresso adds a bold flavor. They can be customized with optional toppings for added indulgence.

Recipe Components:

- 4 oz cream cheese, softened
- 4 oz mascarpone cheese
- 2 tbsps brewed and cooled espresso or strong coffee
- 2 tbsps unsweetened cocoa powder
- 2 tbsps Erythritol or your preferred keto-friendly sweetener
- 1/2 tsp vanilla extract
- 1/4 teacup crushed sugar-free ladyfingers (optional, for covering)
- Unsweetened cocoa powder for dusting (optional)

Preparation Steps: Inside a blending container, blend the softened cream cheese and mascarpone cheese. Mix till smooth and thoroughly mixed. Include the brewed and cooled espresso or coffee, unsweetened cocoa powder, Erythritol (or your sweetener of choice), and vanilla extract to the cheese mixture. Mix till all components are fully incorporated. Line a mini-muffin tin with mini-muffin liners. Scoop the mixture into the muffin liners, filling each around 3/4 full. If desired, mildly dust the tops of the fat bombs with additional unsweetened cocoa powder.

Put the muffin tin in the freezer and let the fat bombs set for almost 2 hrs or till they are firm. If you choose to cover the fat bombs with crushed sugar-free ladyfingers, roll them in the crushed ladyfingers before presenting. Keep the fat bombs in the freezer till you're ready to enjoy them.

Nutritional Info: Calories: 72, Fat: 7g, Protein: 1g, Carb: 2g, Fiber: 1g, Net Carbs: 1g

15. Keto Cinnamon Donut Holes

(Setup Time: 15 mins | Cooked in: 15 mins | 12 donut holes)

Simple to make and requiring minimal setup time, these donut holes are suitable for seniors who enjoy baking but prefer smaller portions. Almond and coconut flours provide fiber and healthy fats. They can be enjoyed as a dessert or snack with a cup of coffee or tea.

Recipe Components:

For the Donut Holes:

- 1 teacup almond flour
- 1/4 teacup coconut flour
- 1/4 teacup granulated Erythritol or your preferred keto-friendly sweetener
- 1 tsp baking powder
- 1/4 tsp salt
- 2 big eggs
- 1/4 teacup unsweetened almond milk
- 1 tsp vanilla extract
- 2 tbsps dissolved coconut oil

For the Cinnamon Coating:

- 2 tbsps granulated Erythritol or your preferred keto-friendly sweetener
- 1 tsp ground cinnamon

Preparation Steps: Warm up your oven to 350 deg.F (175 deg.C) and line a baking sheet with parchment paper. Inside a blending container, blend the almond flour, coconut flour, granulated Erythritol, baking powder, and salt. Mix well. Inside a distinct container, whisk collectively the eggs, unsweetened almond milk, vanilla extract, and dissolved coconut oil. Pour the wet components into the dry components and stir till a dense dough forms. Form the dough into 12 small donut holes and place them on the prepared baking sheet. Bake in the warmed up oven for around 15 mins or till the donut holes are mildly golden. While the donut holes are baking, in a small container, blend collectively the granulated Erythritol and ground cinnamon for the covering. Once the donut holes are done baking, allow them to cool mildly. Then, roll each donut hole in the cinnamon covering mixture till fully covered.

Nutritional Info: Calories: 96, Fat: 7g, Protein: 3g, Carb: 6g, Fiber: 3g, Net Carbs: 3g

16. Espresso Keto Truffles

(Setup Time: 15 mins | Chilling Time: 2h | Approximately 16 truffles)

These truffles offer a rich and intense espresso flavor with a smooth and creamy texture, making them a sophisticated treat for seniors on a ketogenic diet. Unsweetened chocolate provides antioxidants, while espresso adds a caffeine boost.

They can be customized with optional toppings for added flavor and presentation.

Recipe Components:

- 4 oz (115g) unsweetened chocolate, severed
- 2 tbsps unsalted butter
- 2 tbsps strong brewed espresso, cooled
- 1/4 teacup powdered erythritol (or your preferred keto-friendly sweetener)
- 1/2 tsp pure vanilla extract
- 1/8 tsp salt
- Unsweetened cocoa powder (for dusting)
- Optional toppings: crushed espresso beans, unsweetened shredded coconut, or severed nuts

Preparation Steps: Inside a microwave-safe container, blend the severed unsweetened chocolate and butter. Microwave in 20-second intervals, stirring in between, till the chocolate and butter are entirely dissolved and thoroughly mixed. Stir in the brewed espresso, powdered erythritol, vanilla extract, and salt. Mix till the sweetener is dissolved, and the mixture is smooth. Let the mixture cool to room temp. Cover the container and put in the fridge the mixture for around 1-2 hrs or till it firms up but is still pliable. Once the mixture is firm, use a spoon or a small scoop to portion it into approximately 16 truffles. Roll each portion into a ball using your hands. If desired, roll the truffles in unsweetened cocoa powder or your choice of optional toppings. Put the truffles on a parchment-lined tray and return them to the fridge for around 30 mins to set. Serve and enjoy your Espresso Keto Truffles! Store any leftovers in the fridge.

Nutritional Info: Calories: 50, Fat: 5g, Protein: 1g, Carb: 2g, Fiber: 1g, Net Carbs: 1g

---

17. Keto Mixed Berry Parfait

(Setup Time: 10 mins | 2 parfaits)

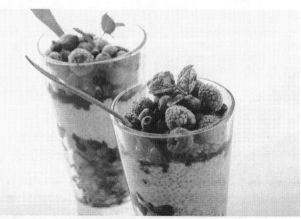

This parfait offers a refreshing combination of mixed berries and creamy yogurt, providing a nutritious and satisfying dessert or snack option for seniors on a ketogenic diet. Greek yogurt adds protein and probiotics, while berries add antioxidants.

Recipe Components:

- 1 teacup fresh mixed berries (e.g., strawberries, blueberries, raspberries)
- 1/2 teacup full-fat Greek yogurt
- 2 tbsps almond butter

- 2 tbsps chia seeds
- 1/2 tsp vanilla extract
- 1-2 tbsps keto-friendly sweetener (adjust as required)
- 1/4 teacup severed nuts (e.g., almonds, walnuts) for topping (optional)

Preparation Steps: Inside a container, mix the full-fat Greek yogurt, almond butter, chia seeds, vanilla extract, and keto-friendly sweetener. Adjust the sweetener to your preferred level of sweetness. Wash and prepare the fresh mixed berries. If the berries are big, consider slicing them into bite-sized pieces. Take two presenting glasses or jars and begin layering your parfait. Start with a spoonful of the yogurt mixture at the bottom. Include a layer of the fresh mixed berries on top of the yogurt mixture. Repeat the layers till the glass is filled, finishing with a layer of berries on top. If desired, spray severed nuts on the very top for added texture and flavor. Chill the parfaits in the fridge for almost 30 mins to allow the chia seeds to denses the yogurt mixture. Serve the Keto Mixed Berry Parfait cold and enjoy!

Nutritional Info: Calories: 320, Fat: 20g, Protein: 12g, Carb: 18g, Fiber: 10g, Net Carbs: 8g

18. Keto Lemon Poppy Seed Muffins

(Setup Time: 10 mins | Cooked in: 25 mins | 12 muffins)

These muffins offer a bright and citrusy flavor with a crunchy poppy seed texture, making them a delightful breakfast or snack option for seniors on a ketogenic diet. Almond flour provides protein and healthy fats. They can be enjoyed warm or at room temperature with a pat of butter or cream cheese.

Recipe Components:

- 2 teacups almond flour
- 1/3 teacup granulated erythritol (or any keto-friendly sweetener)
- 1 1/2 tsps baking powder
- 1 tbsp poppy seeds
- Zest of 2 lemons
- 1/4 teacup fresh lemon juice
- 3 big eggs
- 1/4 teacup unsalted butter, dissolved (or coconut oil for dairy-free)
- 1 tsp vanilla extract

Preparation Steps: Warm up your oven to 350 deg.F (175 deg.C). Line a muffin tin with paper liners or grease it. Inside a big blending container, whisk collectively the almond flour, granulated erythritol, baking powder, and poppy seeds. Inside an extra container, blend the lemon zest, lemon juice, eggs, dissolved butter, and vanilla extract. Pour the wet mixture into the dry mixture and stir till thoroughly mixed. The batter should be dense and smooth. Using a spoon or ice cream scoop, divide the batter evenly among the 12 muffin teacups. Bake in the warmed up oven for around 20-25 mins or till the muffins are golden and a toothpick immersed into the middle comes out clean. Take out the muffins from the oven and allow them to cool in the muffin tin for a couple of mins, then transfer them to a wire stand to cool entirely. Once cooled, enjoy your Keto Lemon Poppy Seed Muffins!

Nutritional Info: Calories: 180, Fat: 15g, Protein: 6g, Carb: 5g, Fiber: 2g, Net Carbs: 3g

19. Cacao Nib and Almond Butter Cups

(Setup Time: 15 mins | Cooked in: 0 mins (refrigeration time required) | 12 teacups)

These cups offer a rich and indulgent chocolate flavor with a creamy almond butter filling, making them a satisfying dessert or snack option for seniors on a ketogenic diet. Cacao nibs provide antioxidants and crunch.

They can be stored in the fridge for easy access and enjoyed throughout the day.

Recipe Components:

- 1/2 teacup cacao nibs
- 1/4 teacup almond butter
- 2 tbsps coconut oil
- 1 tbsp powdered erythritol (or any keto-friendly sweetener)
- A tweak of salt
- 1/2 tsp vanilla extract

Preparation Steps: Inside a microwave-safe container or using a double boiler, dissolve the cacao nibs and coconut oil till smooth. This can be done by microwaving in short intervals or using a double boiler on the stove. Stir in the almond butter, powdered erythritol, salt, and vanilla extract into the dissolved cacao mixture. Mix till the entire components are thoroughly mixed. Line a mini muffin tin with 12 mini muffin liners. Spoon the cacao mixture evenly into each of the 12 teacups. Make sure the bottom is covered. Put the muffin tin in the fridge and let it set for almost 30 mins, or till the teacups are firm. Once set, take out the teacups from the muffin tin and enjoy your Cacao Nib and Almond Butter Cups!

Nutritional Info: Calories: 70, Fat: 6g, Protein: 2g, Carb: 3g, Fiber: 2g, Net Carbs: 1g

20. Keto Cinnamon Pecan Granola

(Setup Time: 10 mins | Cooked in: 25 mins | About 12 presentings)

This granola offers a crunchy texture with a warm cinnamon flavor, making it a satisfying breakfast or snack option for seniors on a ketogenic diet. Almond flour and shredded coconut provide healthy fats and fiber. It can be enjoyed with Greek yogurt or almond milk for added protein and creaminess.

Recipe Components:

- 1 1/2 teacups almond flour
- 1/2 teacup unsweetened shredded coconut
- 1/2 teacup severed pecans
- 1/4 teacup chia seeds
- 1/4 teacup flaxseed meal
- 1/4 teacup erythritol (or any keto-friendly sweetener)
- 1 tsp ground cinnamon
- 1/4 tsp salt
- 1/4 teacup dissolved coconut oil
- 1 big egg
- 1 tsp vanilla extract

Preparation Steps: Warm up your oven to 325 deg.F (160 deg.C) and line a baking sheet with parchment paper. Inside a big blending container, blend the almond flour, shredded coconut, severed pecans, chia seeds, flaxseed meal, erythritol, ground cinnamon, and salt. Inside a distinct container, whisk collectively the dissolved coconut oil, egg, and vanilla extract. Pour the wet mixture over the dry components and stir well till the mixture is evenly covered. Spread the mixture onto the prepared baking sheet and press it down to form an even layer. Bake in the warmed up oven for 20-25 mins or till the granola is golden brown, stirring once halfway through to ensure even cooking. Take out from the oven and let it cool entirely. The granola will become crisp as it cools. Once cooled, break the granola into clusters and store it in a sealed container.

Nutritional Info: Cal: 220, Fat: 19g, Protein: 6g, Carb: 9g, Fiber: 5g, Net Carbs: 4g

90-Day Keto Meal Plan For Seniors

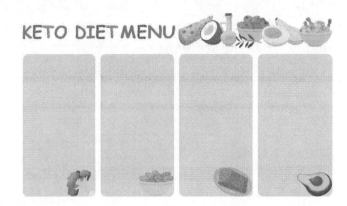

Are you prepared to embark on a transformative journey towards improved health and vitality, tailored specifically for seniors? As a seasoned nutritionist, I have meticulously crafted this 60-day Keto Meal Plan to empower individuals on their ketogenic diet journey. This plan transcends mere weight loss; it embodies a lifestyle that enriches vitality and overall quality of life. It's not a one-size-fits-all solution but rather a meticulously tailored plan for seniors. We recognize the unique needs and challenges faced by individuals as they age, and this plan is designed to address those needs effectively.

Why Follow Our Plan for a Ketogenic Diet?

- ✓ **Optimal Nutrition:** Our meal plan ensures the intake of essential nutrients vital for seniors, including calcium, vitamin D, and B vitamins.

- ✓ **Weight Maintenance:** Aging can pose challenges for weight management, but our plan can aid in maintaining a healthy weight.

- ✓ **Bone Health:** By emphasizing calcium-rich foods, we support bone health and reduce the risk of osteoporosis.

- ✓ **Heart Health:** A well-structured ketogenic diet can promote cardiovascular health, crucial as individuals age.

- ✓ **Enhanced Cognitive Function:** The balanced ketogenic diet provides a consistent energy supply to the brain, essential for maintaining cognitive function. Foods rich in healthy fats and antioxidants may support memory, mental clarity, and overall brain health as individuals age.

- ✓ **Improved Digestive Health:** Age-related digestive changes can lead to issues like constipation or nutrient malabsorption. Our plan includes foods gentle on the digestive system, such as fiber-rich vegetables and probiotic-rich options like yogurt or sauerkraut, promoting gut health and regularity.

- ✓ **Blood Sugar Control:** The ketogenic diet aids in regulating blood sugar levels, vital for older adults to reduce the risk of diabetes and support overall well-being.

- ✓ **Reduced Inflammation:** Inflammation is linked to various age-related conditions like arthritis and cardiovascular diseases. The anti-inflammatory properties of many foods in our meal plan, like fatty fish and leafy greens, can help reduce inflammation, promoting joint and heart health.

✓ **Increased Energy Levels:** Many seniors experience a decline in energy levels. The ketogenic diet's emphasis on healthy fats as an energy source provides a sustainable and steady energy supply, combating feelings of fatigue.

✓ **Hormonal Balance:** Hormonal changes are common as individuals age. Our meal plan includes foods that support hormonal balance, such as those rich in omega-3 fatty acids and antioxidants, aiding in managing symptoms associated with menopause and aging.

✓ **Enhanced Skin Health:** A diet rich in antioxidants and healthy fats can support skin health and combat signs of aging. Our plan comprises foods like avocados and berries, which are known for their skin benefits.

Day 1	Day 2
Breakfast: Creamy Avocado and Smoked Salmon Toast	Breakfast: Blueberry Chia Pudding
Lunch: Keto Chicken and Vegetable Stir-Fry	Lunch: Spinach and Feta Stuffed Chicken Breast
Dinner: Creamy Spinach and Mushroom Stuffed Pork Tenderloin	Dinner: Keto Eggplant Lasagna
Snack: Coconut Almond Butter Bites	Snack: Pumpkin Spice Keto Cookies
Day 3	Day 4
Breakfast: Spinach and Mushroom Breakfast Casserole	Breakfast: Cauliflower Hash Browns
Lunch: Greek-inspired Cucumber and Tomato Salad	Lunch: Zucchini Noodles with Pesto and Cherry Tomatoes
Dinner: Dijon and Herb Crusted Salmon	Dinner: Keto Beef Stroganoff
Snack: Matcha Green Tea Fat Bombs	Snack: Keto Peanut Butter Fudge
Day 5	Day 6
Breakfast: Coconut Almond Keto Pancakes	Breakfast: Cheddar and Chive Keto Biscuits
Lunch: Keto Beef and Broccoli	Lunch: Baked Cod with Lemon and Dill
Dinner: Lemon Garlic Shrimp and Zucchini Noodles	Dinner: Spicy Cauliflower and Chickpea Curry
Snack: Blueberry Almond Keto Granola	Snack: Chocolate Mint Avocado Pudding

Day 7	Day 8
Breakfast: Turmeric Scrambled Eggs	Breakfast: Keto Strawberry Smoothie Bowl
Lunch: Asparagus and Prosciutto Wraps	Lunch: Eggplant Parmesan
Dinner: Pesto and Prosciutto-Wrapped Asparagus	Dinner: Lemon Butter Baked Cod with Herbed Tomatoes
Snack: Cinnamon Pecan Keto Brittle	Snack: Cinnamon Pecan Keto Brittle
Day 9	Day 10
Breakfast: Bacon-Wrapped Asparagus	Breakfast: Almond Flour Waffles
Lunch: Shrimp and Cauliflower Rice Stir-Fry	Lunch: Cauliflower and Bacon Soup
Dinner: Stuffed Zucchini Boats with Ground Turkey	Dinner: Creamy Spinach and Artichoke Stuffed Chicken Breasts
Snack: Keto Cheesecake Bites	Snack: Peanut Butter Chocolate Chip Keto Bars
Day 11	Day 12
Breakfast: Tomato and Basil Mini Quiches	Breakfast: Mediterranean Keto Omelette
Lunch: Avocado and Tuna Stuffed Bell Peppers	Lunch: Keto Turkey and Cranberry Salad
Dinner: Roasted Garlic and Rosemary Lamb Chops	Dinner: Thai-inspired Coconut Shrimp Soup
Snack: Salted Caramel Fat Bombs	Snack: Chocolate Dipped Macadamia Nut Bites
Day 13	Day 14
Breakfast: Keto Veggie and Cheese Frittata Muffins	Breakfast: Cinnamon Coconut Porridge
Lunch: Keto Cabbage Rolls	Lunch: Thai-inspired Coconut Shrimp Soup
Dinner: Keto Spaghetti Squash Carbonara	Dinner: Baked Dijon Mustard and Herb-Crusted Tilapia
Snack: Coconut Lime Energy Bites	Snack: Keto Tiramisu Fat Bombs

Day 15	Day 16
Breakfast: Savory Keto Crepes	Breakfast: Pecan Pie Keto Oatmeal
Lunch: Spinach and Mushroom Stuffed Pork Chops	Lunch: Creamy Garlic Shrimp with Spinach
Dinner: Cabbage and Sausage Stir-Fry	Dinner: Keto Pork Chops with Blue Cheese Sauce
Snack: Keto Cinnamon Donut Holes	Snack: Espresso Keto Truffles
Day 17	Day 18
Breakfast: Coconut Berry Parfait	Breakfast: Keto Zucchini Bread
Lunch: Greek Lemon Chicken Soup (Avgolemono Soup)	Lunch: Keto BLT Salad
Dinner: Keto Pesto and Mozzarella Stuffed Chicken	Dinner: Lemon Herb Shrimp and Zucchini Noodles
Snack: Keto Mixed Berry Parfait	Snack: Keto Lemon Poppy Seed Muffins
Day 19	Day 20
Breakfast: Keto Cinnamon Roll Chaffles	Breakfast: Greek Yogurt and Walnut Parfait
Lunch: Spinach and Artichoke Stuffed Chicken	Lunch: Salmon and Avocado Salad
Dinner: Beef and Broccoli Stir-Fry with Sesame Seeds	Dinner: Stuffed Avocado with Tuna and Olive Tapenade
Snack: Keto Cinnamon Pecan Granola	Snack: Cacao Nib and Almond Butter Cups
Day 21	Day 22
Breakfast: Keto Strawberry Smoothie Bowl	Breakfast: Bacon-Wrapped Asparagus
Lunch: Keto Turkey and Cranberry Salad	Lunch: Keto Cabbage Rolls
Dinner: Lemon Garlic Shrimp and Zucchini Noodles	Dinner: Spicy Cauliflower and Chickpea Curry
Snack: Keto Cheesecake Bites	Snack: Peanut Butter Chocolate Chip Keto Bars

Day 23	Day 24
Breakfast: Tomato and Basil Mini Quiches	Breakfast: Coconut Almond Keto Pancakes
Lunch: Thai Coconut Chicken Soup	Lunch: Spinach and Mushroom Stuffed Pork Chops
Dinner: Pesto and Prosciutto-Wrapped Asparagus	Dinner: Lemon Butter Baked Cod with Herbed Tomatoes
Snack: Salted Caramel Fat Bombs	Snack: Chocolate Dipped Macadamia Nut Bites
Day 25	**Day 26**
Breakfast: Blueberry Chia Pudding	Breakfast: Mediterranean Keto Omelette
Lunch: Creamy Garlic Shrimp with Spinach	Lunch: Greek Lemon Chicken Soup (Avgolemono Soup)
Dinner: Stuffed Zucchini Boats with Ground Turkey	Dinner: Creamy Spinach and Artichoke Stuffed Chicken Breasts
Snack: Coconut Lime Energy Bites	Snack: Keto Tiramisu Fat Bombs
Day 27	**Day 28**
Breakfast: Cinnamon Coconut Porridge	Breakfast: Keto Veggie and Cheese Frittata Muffins
Lunch: Keto BLT Salad	Lunch: Spinach and Artichoke Stuffed Chicken
Dinner: Roasted Garlic and Rosemary Lamb Chops	Dinner: Thai-inspired Coconut Shrimp Soup
Snack: Keto Cinnamon Donut Holes	Snack: Espresso Keto Truffles
Day 29	**Day 30**
Breakfast: Pecan Pie Keto Oatmeal	Breakfast: Coconut Berry Parfait
Lunch: Salmon and Avocado Salad	Lunch: Creamy Spinach and Mushroom Stuffed Pork Tenderloin
Dinner: Keto Spaghetti Squash Carbonara	Dinner: Baked Dijon Mustard and Herb-Crusted Tilapia

Snack: Keto Mixed Berry Parfait	Snack: Keto Lemon Poppy Seed Muffins
Day 31	**Day 32**
Breakfast: Blueberry Almond Keto Granola	Breakfast: Keto Cinnamon Roll Chaffles
Lunch: Cabbage and Sausage Stir-Fry	Lunch: Thai Coconut Chicken Soup
Dinner: Keto Pork Chops with Blue Cheese Sauce	Dinner: Stuffed Zucchini Boats with Ground Turkey
Snack: Chocolate Dipped Macadamia Nut Bites	Snack: Keto Cheesecake Bites
Day 33	**Day 34**
Breakfast: Savory Keto Crepes	Breakfast: Coconut Almond Keto Pancakes
Lunch: Spinach and Mushroom Stuffed Pork Chops	Lunch: Greek-inspired Cucumber and Tomato Salad
Dinner: Creamy Spinach and Artichoke Stuffed Chicken Breasts	Dinner: Pesto and Prosciutto-Wrapped Asparagus
Snack: Peanut Butter Chocolate Chip Keto Bars	Snack: Salted Caramel Fat Bombs
Day 35	**Day 36**
Breakfast: Bacon-Wrapped Asparagus	Breakfast: Keto Strawberry Smoothie Bowl
Lunch: Zucchini Noodles with Pesto and Cherry Tomatoes	Lunch: Keto Beef and Broccoli
Dinner: Lemon Butter Baked Cod with Herbed Tomatoes	Dinner: Stuffed Avocado with Tuna and Olive Tapenade
Snack: Chocolate Dipped Macadamia Nut Bites	Snack: Keto Tiramisu Fat Bombs
Day 37	**Day 38**
Breakfast: Mediterranean Keto Omelette	Breakfast: Keto Veggie and Cheese Frittata Muffins
Lunch: Asparagus and Prosciutto Wraps	Lunch: Eggplant Parmesan

Dinner: Beef and Broccoli Stir-Fry with Sesame Seeds	Dinner: Keto Spaghetti Squash Carbonara
Snack: Cacao Nib and Almond Butter Cups	Snack: Keto Peanut Butter Fudge
Day 39	**Day 40**
Breakfast: Cinnamon Coconut Porridge	Breakfast: Almond Flour Waffles
Lunch: Shrimp and Cauliflower Rice Stir-Fry	Lunch: Cauliflower and Bacon Soup
Dinner: Baked Dijon Mustard and Herb-Crusted Tilapia	Dinner: Cabbage and Sausage Stir-Fry
Snack: Coconut Almond Butter Bites	Snack: Pumpkin Spice Keto Cookies
Day 41	**Day 42**
Breakfast: Tomato and Basil Mini Quiches	Breakfast: Creamy Avocado and Smoked Salmon Toast
Lunch: Avocado and Tuna Stuffed Bell Peppers	Lunch: Keto Turkey and Cranberry Salad
Dinner: Keto Pork Chops with Blue Cheese Sauce	Dinner: Lemon Garlic Shrimp and Zucchini Noodles
Snack: Blueberry Almond Keto Granola	Snack: Matcha Green Tea Fat Bombs
Day 43	**Day 44**
Breakfast: Spinach and Mushroom Breakfast Casserole	Breakfast: Cauliflower Hash Browns
Lunch: Keto Cabbage Rolls	Lunch: Thai Coconut Chicken Soup
Dinner: Spicy Cauliflower and Chickpea Curry	Dinner: Pesto and Prosciutto-Wrapped Asparagus
Snack: Keto Cheesecake Bites	Snack: Peanut Butter Chocolate Chip Keto Bars
Day 45	**Day 46**
Breakfast: Cheddar and Chive Keto Biscuits	Breakfast: Turmeric Scrambled Eggs

Lunch: Spinach and Artichoke Stuffed Chicken	Lunch: Salmon and Avocado Salad
Dinner: Lemon Herb Shrimp and Zucchini Noodles	Dinner: Stuffed Avocado with Tuna and Olive Tapenade
Snack: Salted Caramel Fat Bombs	Snack: Chocolate Dipped Macadamia Nut Bites
Day 47	**Day 48**
Breakfast: Keto Strawberry Smoothie Bowl	Breakfast: Bacon-Wrapped Asparagus
Lunch: Creamy Spinach and Mushroom Stuffed Pork Tenderloin	Lunch: Keto Eggplant Lasagna
Dinner: Keto Beef Stroganoff	Dinner: Lemon Butter Baked Cod with Herbed Tomatoes
Snack: Coconut Lime Energy Bites	Snack: Keto Tiramisu Fat Bombs
Day 49	**Day 50**
Breakfast: Almond Flour Waffles	Breakfast: Tomato and Basil Mini Quiches
Lunch: Dijon and Herb Crusted Salmon	Lunch: Keto Spaghetti Squash Carbonara
Dinner: Stuffed Zucchini Boats with Ground Turkey	Dinner: Creamy Spinach and Artichoke Stuffed Chicken Breasts
Snack: Keto Mixed Berry Parfait	Snack: Keto Lemon Poppy Seed Muffins
Day 51	**Day 52**
Breakfast: Spinach and Mushroom Breakfast Casserole	Breakfast: Pecan Pie Keto Oatmeal
Lunch: Baked Dijon Mustard and Herb-Crusted Tilapia	Lunch: Cabbage and Sausage Stir-Fry
Dinner: Roasted Garlic and Rosemary Lamb Chops	Dinner: Thai-inspired Coconut Shrimp Soup
Snack: Keto Cinnamon Donut Holes	Snack: Espresso Keto Truffles

Day 53	Day 54
Breakfast: Coconut Berry Parfait	Breakfast: Keto Zucchini Bread
Lunch: Keto Pork Chops with Blue Cheese Sauce	Lunch: Lemon Herb Shrimp and Zucchini Noodles
Dinner: Keto Pesto and Mozzarella Stuffed Chicken	Dinner: Lemon Garlic Shrimp and Zucchini Noodles
Snack: Keto Cinnamon Pecan Granola	Snack: Coconut Almond Butter Bites
Day 55	Day 56
Breakfast: Keto Cinnamon Roll Chaffles	Breakfast: Greek Yogurt and Walnut Parfait
Lunch: Beef and Broccoli Stir-Fry with Sesame Seeds	Lunch: Spinach and Artichoke Stuffed Chicken
Dinner: Stuffed Avocado with Tuna and Olive Tapenade	Dinner: Creamy Spinach and Mushroom Stuffed Pork Tenderloin
Snack: Pumpkin Spice Keto Cookies	Snack: Chocolate Mint Avocado Pudding
Day 57	Day 58
Breakfast: Creamy Avocado and Smoked Salmon Toast	Breakfast: Keto Veggie and Cheese Frittata Muffins
Lunch: Salmon and Avocado Salad	Lunch: Creamy Spinach and Artichoke Stuffed Chicken Breasts
Dinner: Keto Beef Stroganoff	Dinner: Lemon Butter Baked Cod with Herbed Tomatoes
Snack: Cacao Nib and Almond Butter Cups	Snack: Keto Peanut Butter Fudge
Day 59	Day 60
Breakfast: Cinnamon Coconut Porridge	Breakfast: Blueberry Chia Pudding
Lunch: Shrimp and Cauliflower Rice Stir-Fry	Lunch: Thai Coconut Chicken Soup
Dinner: Stuffed Zucchini Boats with Ground Turkey	Dinner: Keto Pesto and Mozzarella Stuffed Chicken

Snack: Coconut Lime Energy Bites	Snack: Keto Cheesecake Bites
Day 61	**Day 62**
Breakfast: Turmeric Scrambled Eggs	Breakfast: Cauliflower Hash Browns
Lunch: Keto Cabbage Rolls	Lunch: Thai Coconut Chicken Soup
Dinner: Lemon Garlic Shrimp and Zucchini Noodles	Dinner: Pesto and Prosciutto-Wrapped Asparagus
Snack: Matcha Green Tea Fat Bombs	Snack: Peanut Butter Chocolate Chip Keto Bars
Day 63	**Day 64**
Breakfast: Cheddar and Chive Keto Biscuits	Breakfast: Savory Keto Crepes
Lunch: Spinach and Artichoke Stuffed Chicken	Lunch: Salmon and Avocado Salad
Dinner: Lemon Herb Shrimp and Zucchini Noodles	Dinner: Stuffed Avocado with Tuna and Olive Tapenade
Snack: Salted Caramel Fat Bombs	Snack: Chocolate Dipped Macadamia Nut Bites
Day 65	**Day 66**
Breakfast: Keto Strawberry Smoothie Bowl	Breakfast: Bacon-Wrapped Asparagus
Lunch: Creamy Spinach and Mushroom Stuffed Pork Tenderloin	Lunch: Keto Eggplant Lasagna
Dinner: Keto Beef Stroganoff	Dinner: Lemon Butter Baked Cod with Herbed Tomatoes
Snack: Coconut Lime Energy Bites	Snack: Keto Tiramisu Fat Bombs
Day 67	**Day 68**
Breakfast: Almond Flour Waffles	Breakfast: Tomato and Basil Mini Quiches
Lunch: Dijon and Herb Crusted Salmon	Lunch: Keto Spaghetti Squash Carbonara

Dinner: Stuffed Zucchini Boats with Ground Turkey	Dinner: Creamy Spinach and Artichoke Stuffed Chicken Breasts
Snack: Keto Mixed Berry Parfait	Snack: Keto Lemon Poppy Seed Muffins
Day 69	**Day 70**
Breakfast: Spinach and Mushroom Breakfast Casserole	Breakfast: Pecan Pie Keto Oatmeal
Lunch: Baked Dijon Mustard and Herb-Crusted Tilapia	Lunch: Cabbage and Sausage Stir-Fry
Dinner: Roasted Garlic and Rosemary Lamb Chops	Dinner: Thai-inspired Coconut Shrimp Soup
Snack: Keto Cinnamon Donut Holes	Snack: Espresso Keto Truffles
Day 71	**Day 72**
Breakfast: Coconut Berry Parfait	Breakfast: Keto Zucchini Bread
Lunch: Keto Pork Chops with Blue Cheese Sauce	Lunch: Lemon Herb Shrimp and Zucchini Noodles
Dinner: Keto Pesto and Mozzarella Stuffed Chicken	Dinner: Lemon Garlic Shrimp and Zucchini Noodles
Snack: Keto Cinnamon Pecan Granola	Snack: Coconut Almond Butter Bites
Day 73	**Day 74**
Breakfast: Keto Cinnamon Roll Chaffles	Breakfast: Greek Yogurt and Walnut Parfait
Lunch: Beef and Broccoli Stir-Fry with Sesame Seeds	Lunch: Spinach and Artichoke Stuffed Chicken
Dinner: Stuffed Avocado with Tuna and Olive Tapenade	Dinner: Creamy Spinach and Mushroom Stuffed Pork Tenderloin
Snack: Pumpkin Spice Keto Cookies	Snack: Chocolate Mint Avocado Pudding

Day 75	Day 76
Breakfast: Creamy Avocado and Smoked Salmon Toast	Breakfast: Keto Veggie and Cheese Frittata Muffins
Lunch: Salmon and Avocado Salad	Lunch: Creamy Spinach and Artichoke Stuffed Chicken Breasts
Dinner: Keto Beef Stroganoff	Dinner: Lemon Butter Baked Cod with Herbed Tomatoes
Snack: Cacao Nib and Almond Butter Cups	Snack: Keto Peanut Butter Fudge
Day 77	Day 78
Breakfast: Cinnamon Coconut Porridge	Breakfast: Blueberry Chia Pudding
Lunch: Shrimp and Cauliflower Rice Stir-Fry	Lunch: Thai Coconut Chicken Soup
Dinner: Stuffed Zucchini Boats with Ground Turkey	Dinner: Keto Pesto and Mozzarella Stuffed Chicken
Snack: Coconut Lime Energy Bites	Snack: Keto Cheesecake Bites
Day 79	Day 80
Breakfast: Turmeric Scrambled Eggs	Breakfast: Cauliflower Hash Browns
Lunch: Keto Cabbage Rolls	Lunch: Thai Coconut Chicken Soup
Dinner: Lemon Garlic Shrimp and Zucchini Noodles	Dinner: Pesto and Prosciutto-Wrapped Asparagus
Snack: Matcha Green Tea Fat Bombs	Snack: Peanut Butter Chocolate Chip Keto Bar
Day 81	Day 82
Breakfast: Cheddar and Chive Keto Biscuits	Breakfast: Savory Keto Crepes
Lunch: Spinach and Artichoke Stuffed Chicken	Lunch: Salmon and Avocado Salad
Dinner: Lemon Herb Shrimp and Zucchini Noodles	Dinner: Stuffed Avocado with Tuna and Olive Tapenade

Snack: Salted Caramel Fat Bombs	Snack: Chocolate Dipped Macadamia Nut Bites
Day 83	**Day 84**
Breakfast: Keto Strawberry Smoothie Bowl	Breakfast: Bacon-Wrapped Asparagus
Lunch: Creamy Spinach and Mushroom Stuffed Pork Tenderloin	Lunch: Keto Eggplant Lasagna
Dinner: Keto Beef Stroganoff	Dinner: Lemon Butter Baked Cod with Herbed Tomatoes
Snack: Coconut Lime Energy Bites	Snack: Keto Tiramisu Fat Bombs
Day 85	**Day 86**
Breakfast: Almond Flour Waffles	Breakfast: Tomato and Basil Mini Quiches
Lunch: Dijon and Herb Crusted Salmon	Lunch: Keto Spaghetti Squash Carbonara
Dinner: Stuffed Zucchini Boats with Ground Turkey	Dinner: Creamy Spinach and Artichoke Stuffed Chicken Breasts
Snack: Keto Mixed Berry Parfait	Snack: Keto Lemon Poppy Seed Muffins
Day 87	**Day 88**
Breakfast: Spinach and Mushroom Breakfast Casserole	Breakfast: Pecan Pie Keto Oatmeal
Lunch: Baked Dijon Mustard and Herb-Crusted Tilapia	Lunch: Cabbage and Sausage Stir-Fry
Dinner: Roasted Garlic and Rosemary Lamb Chops	Dinner: Thai-inspired Coconut Shrimp Soup
Snack: Keto Cinnamon Donut Holes	Snack: Espresso Keto Truffles
Day 89	**Day 90**
Breakfast: Coconut Berry Parfait	Breakfast: Keto Zucchini Bread
Lunch: Keto Pork Chops with Blue Cheese Sauce	Lunch: Lemon Herb Shrimp and Zucchini Noodles
Dinner: Keto Pesto and Mozzarella Stuffed	Dinner: Lemon Garlic Shrimp and Zucchini

Chicken	Noodles
Snack: Keto Cinnamon Pecan Granola	Snack: Coconut Almond Butter Bites

Congratulations On Completing The 90-Day Keto Meal Plan!

By now, you should have acclimated to this dietary regimen and felt its potential advantages. Keep in mind to continue making mindful dietary decisions and heeding your body's requirements.

Below, we've summarized helpful suggestions covered throughout our book tailored specifically for seniors:

- ✓ **Stay Hydrated:** Aging may diminish the sensation of thirst, so make a conscious effort to consume an adequate amount of water daily.

- ✓ **Maintain Muscle Mass:** Engaging in regular exercise, particularly strength training, can assist in preserving muscle mass and strength.

- ✓ **Monitor Bone Health:** Regular check-ups for bone density and supplementation when necessary are imperative for maintaining healthy bones.

- ✓ **Mindful Eating:** Be mindful of portion sizes and avoid unnecessary snacking.

- ✓ **Consult a Healthcare Professional:** Before implementing significant dietary changes, it's advisable to consult with a healthcare provider, especially if you have pre-existing health conditions.

- ✓ **Grocery Shopping:** Choose fresh, whole foods, and prioritize organic and locally sourced options when available.

- ✓ **Listen to Your Body:** Nutritional requirements may shift with age, so pay attention to your body's cues and make adjustments as needed.

- ✓ **Social Connection:** Nurturing social connections and remaining engaged with loved ones is essential for emotional well-being.

- ✓ **Regular Health Screenings:** Schedule routine check-ups to detect and address health concerns early, including eye and dental examinations.

- ✓ **Mental Wellness:** Prioritize mental well-being through practices such as meditation, mindfulness, or engaging in enjoyable hobbies.

- ✓ **Quality Sleep:** Ensure you obtain adequate and restorative sleep to support overall health and vitality.

- ✓ **Eye Health:** Regular eye examinations are crucial as eye health can decline with age. Consider incorporating foods rich in lutein and zeaxanthin, such as leafy greens, to promote optimal eye health.

Keto Diet for Seniors Guided Nutrition Tracker

Name:

Start Date of Tracking:

Keto Diet Goal:

Ketosis Level:

Monitor and record your ketosis level daily using keto test strips.

Day 1	Day 2
Ketosis Level:	Ketosis Level:
Notes:	Notes:

...

Nutrition Intake

Log the meals and snacks you consume. Pay attention to portion sizes and the quality of foods you choose.

Day 1

Meal 1:

Meal 2:

Snack:

Meal 3:

Notes:

Day 2

Meal 1:

Meal 2:

Snack:

Meal 3:

Notes:

...

Non-Scale Victories

Every day, write down the non-scale victories you experienced thanks to the ketogenic diet. These could include improved digestion, reduced cravings, enhanced focus, or healthier skin.

Day 1

Non-Scale Victory:

Notes:

...

Day 2

Non-Scale Victory:

Notes:

Energy and Well-being

Monitor your energy levels and overall well-being throughout the day. Take note of any variations or changes you noticed.

Day 1

Energy Levels:

General Well-being:

Notes:

Day 2

Energy Levels:

General Well-being:

Notes:

...

Physical Changes

Occasionally, take time to evaluate any physical changes related to the ketogenic diet. These may include changes in weight, measurements, or body composition.

Day 1

Weight:

Measurements:

Body Composition:

Notes:

Day 2

Weight:

Measurements:

Body Composition:

Notes:

...

Guided Roadmap for the Keto Diet

These guidelines will assist you in tracking your progress on the ketogenic diet in a structured and mindful manner. Exercise patience with yourself, as responses may differ from person to person. Customize the keto diet to meet your specific requirements and experiment until you discover the optimal routine for your journey.

Step 1: Select Your Tracking Method

Choose the tracking method that aligns with your preferences: traditional pen and paper, a mobile app, or a smartwatch/fitness tracker.

Step 2: Establish Clear Objectives

Clearly outline your keto diet objectives, such as attaining and sustaining ketosis, managing weight, increasing energy levels, or enhancing mental clarity.

Step 3: Monitoring Ketosis Levels

Regularly measure and track your ketosis levels using keto test strips to ensure you're consistently in a state of ketosis.

Step 4: Mindful Eating

Monitor your food intake, prioritizing nutritious and balanced choices in line with the Keto Diet.

Step 5: Acknowledge Non-Scale Achievements

Recognize achievements unrelated to weight, such as improved sleep quality, reduced inflammation, or enhanced mood.

Step 6: Awareness of Energy and Well-being

Stay attuned to your energy levels throughout the day and observe how the ketogenic diet influences your overall well-being.

Step 7: Assessing Physical Transformations

Periodically evaluate any physical changes, bearing in mind that progress may be gradual and vary between individuals.

Step 8: Reflection and Adjustment

On a weekly basis, reflect on your progress and adjust your ketogenic diet regimen based on outcomes and personal requirements.

Step 9: Celebrate Success

Celebrate both significant milestones and small victories along your ketogenic diet journey to maintain high levels of motivation.

Conclusion

As we conclude this journey through the world of the ketogenic diet, it's essential to reflect on the key concepts and insights we've explored together. The path to healthy aging is marked by choices, and adopting the ketogenic lifestyle can be transformative.

Throughout this book, we've examined the natural changes that occur in our bodies as we age and how the ketogenic diet can play a crucial role in promoting graceful aging. We've discussed achieving and maintaining ketosis safely, as well as the different variations of the ketogenic diet that can be tailored to meet the unique needs of seniors. Balancing diet with lifestyle, overcoming challenges, and addressing potential risks and side effects have been central themes.

The benefits of the ketogenic diet for seniors are significant. From supporting bone health to enhancing heart health, this lifestyle choice can truly improve quality of life. It empowers us to maintain a healthy weight, preserve muscle mass, and ensure optimal nutrition.

I encourage every senior to embark on this ketogenic journey with enthusiasm and care. The advantages for health and well-being are clear, and you are not alone in this endeavor. Many seniors worldwide have embraced this lifestyle, forming a supportive community that celebrates the joys of healthy aging through the ketogenic diet.

With mindful eating, regular exercise, and the guidance provided in this book, you are equipped to embrace the ketogenic diet and its remarkable potential. The path to a healthier, more vibrant you starts here, with the benefits awaiting your embrace. Embrace this transformative journey, and may it bring you health, vitality, and the joy of aging gracefully.

Dear Reader,

Thank you for taking the time to explore "Keto Diet For Seniors". As the author, I'm deeply passionate about empowering individuals to take control of their health through mindful eating and balanced nutrition.

Your feedback is incredibly valuable, not only to me but also to other potential readers who are considering this book. By sharing your thoughts and experiences, you're not only helping me improve as an author but also assisting others in making informed decisions about their health journey.

I kindly invite you to leave a review on the Amazon website. Your review can provide insight and guidance to those who may benefit from the information shared in this book. Whether you found the recipes helpful, the information enlightening, or have suggestions for improvement, your feedback matters.

Leaving a review is simple. Just scan the QR code below with your mobile phone, and it will take you directly to the review page on Amazon. Your honest review will make a difference, and I'm grateful for your support in spreading the message of health and well-being.

Thank you for being a part of this journey.

Warm regards,
Melinda Francis

Made in the USA
Las Vegas, NV
13 April 2024